DO NOT REMOVE
CARDS FROM POCKET

Breast Care
Options
For the 1990's

Breast Care
Options
For the 1990's

Paul Kuehn, M.D.

Newmark Publishing Company

Published by Newmark Publishing Company
South Windsor, CT 06074
(203)282-7265

Designed by Irving Perkins Associates, Inc.
Typeset by Pagesetters Incorporated
Printed and Bound by The Book Press
Manufactured in the United States of America

10   9   8   7   6   5   4   3   2   1

Library of Congress Cataloging in Publication Data

Kuehn, Paul
Breast Care Options for the 1990's
1. Risk Factors   2. Limited Surgery vs. Mastectomy   3. Stress, Diet
4. Brittle Bones

91–060345

ISBN 0–938539–04–3

Contents

Introduction

In 1986, Dr. Paul Kuehn, a cancer surgeon, wrote *Breast Care Options*. This popular book was universally accepted by the reading public and libraries as an important reference for up-to-date advancements in the diagnosis and treatment of breast disease. It was written primarily for the woman who wished to be informed prior to giving consent to treatment. The highly successful first edition was selected by *Prevention Magazine* for its book club. The book was also translated into Spanish for international distribution.

This new book has been completely revised. Nine new chapters have been added, including one on needle localization of non-palpable breast tumors. Dr. Kuehn also discusses controversies concerning the treatment of tiny breast cancers such as intraductal cancer and lobular carcinoma in situ.

As experience is gained in diagnostic mammography, minimal cancers are being detected and breast conservation methods utilized more often. One chapter compares the results of limited surgery with those of mastectomy and discusses the pros and cons of each method. Not all patients qualify for limited surgery, and many have experienced spread of their cancer when first diagnosed.

In recent statistics published by the National Cancer Institute, the incidence of cancer of the breast in both white and black women is higher today than for any other year since 1973. This is true for any age group. The disease, it seems, has not been conquered; innovative research must continue in order to find a cure.

Attempts at prevention—such as the right diet and steady exercise—are helpful, and new diagnostic methods such as mammography and ultrasound are aiding in detection. Stereotaxic needle biopsy of breast tumors may eventually eliminate the need for open biopsy in diagnosing unusual breast changes. Further, the role that genetics play in breast disease is being clarified. Flow cytometry may define those patients who are at greater risk, so that treatment such as chemotherapy may be administered more intelligently.

Biopsy of the glands under the arm on the side of the malignant breast tumor, whether a lumpectomy or mastectomy, is now regularly performed to determine whether the tumor has spread. In some centers, this is no longer being done for tiny minimal cancers, as new, non-invasive methods are developed to help avoid this procedure.

The care of the second breast after discovery and treatment of cancer in the first breast is controversial. You'll find this issue discussed in a completely new chapter.

There have been numerous new discoveries and advancements since the publication of *Breast Care Options*. This new book will help the woman with a breast problem to review new methods of detection and participate more fully in her treatment—for the 1990's.

Breast Care
Options
For the 1990's

1

The Disease Women Fear Most

The incidence of breast cancer continues to rise in the United States for both white and black women. This is true for those both under and over 50 years of age. Breast cancer, in fact, is one of the major medical problems for women in this country. While progress has been made, 150,000 new cases of breast cancer are diagnosed each year and 50,000 women are dying of the disease each year. One in nine women will develop breast cancer during her normal life expectancy.

In the past, good screening methods were not readily available and diagnostic tools were limited. As a result, most women detected the cancers in their breasts by breast self-examination. Treatment methods were primitive and, if there was no evidence of the cancer spreading, radical mastectomy was usually performed. Yet 50 percent of patients did show evidence of spreading cancer when it was first detected.[1,2] Radiation therapy was given, attempts at chemotherapy were instituted, and both were usually unsuccessful.

Luckily, the dogma of radical surgery for most cases was successfully challenged so that today a woman often qualifies for limited surgery to save her breast. The accompanying psychological trauma, as well as the

1

physical and cosmetic consequences, have been reduced. Many women who have been able to avoid radical surgery have survived and thrived both physiologically and emotionally.

Combined diagnostic and treatment methods used today have recently evolved to a point where surgical oncologists, radiation therapists, and medical oncologists can reach a consensus as to the best treatment for each patient. Much of this substantial progress has been achieved during the years since *Breast Care Options* was published. The acceptance of screening methods has been accelerated and up-front. Aggressive, primary, adjuvant, systemic therapy has been advocated. During the past ten years, breast cancer five-year survival rates have increased only 5 percent. The survival rate today is 74 percent. Mortality rates, however, have remained the same,[3,4] suggesting that our diagnostic methods have improved (mammography), but our treatment methods have not.

The acceptance of mammography as a diagnostic tool to detect tiny nonpalpable tumors has led to the increased use of limited surgery to save the breast.

Modified mastectomy, combined with axillary node dissection to determine spread of the disease, is still used in many cases, if there is suspected diffuse involvement of the breast (multicentricity). Attempts are being made to define those women who are at high risk for recurrence and to determine who should undergo mastectomy and who qualifies for limited surgery.

Breast cancer is a disease apparently influenced by many factors—age, heredity, childbearing, hormones, socioeconomic status, drugs, stress, and—according to some authorities—a diet high in fats. None of the suspected causes, however, explain fully why breast cancer is on the increase in this country.

There has been considerable controversy as to whether breast cancer originates from a single cell that goes haywire and then multiplies, invades tissue, and spreads to vital organs, or is a systemic disease from its onset.[5] The concept of radical surgery was to cut out the cancer in its entirety before it spread. Radiation therapy was given after surgery to "mop up" by destroying any remaining cancerous cells, and to make the patient cancer-free. Neither of these methods worked completely. Chemotherapy was then given to introduce cancerocidal drugs into the bloodstream and lymphatics to try to kill any free-floating cancer cells. The first chemotherapeutic drugs were very toxic and caused serious side effects. New drugs and combinations of drugs have been more successful and the methods of administration varied to reduce the effects of toxicity.

There are scientists who still feel that breast cancer is not a systemic disease. They point out that even with the old-fashioned method of radical mastectomy, as many as half of the women who underwent it survived five years. Many of those patients lived for more than 25 years and died of other causes. If breast cancer is to be theorized as a systemic disease, how did these patients survive?

In the forefront of the war against breast cancer, methods of prevention have not been emphasized. Diets in this country generally center on simplistic methods of satisfying appetites. All one has to do is look at the success and alarming proliferation of the fast-food restaurants where meals resplendent in fatty acids are served. Obesity created by food is often a precursor to breast cancer. Vegetarians, for instance, show a low incidence of breast cancer, and in countries where beef consumption is low (Japan, for instance) the incidence of breast cancer is much lower. Moreover, a high-fat, low-fiber diet definitely increases the risk for breast cancer.[6]

The relationship between cholesterol levels and heart disease has recently been showcased by the news media. Medication to reduce cholesterol levels and eating cereals high in fiber content have been stressed as methods for keeping cholesterol levels low. With the deluge of statistics came this fact: the average consumption of animal fat (triglycerides) in this country is much too high; it accounts for 40 percent of our total caloric intake. This has to be reduced, and the consumption of fiber must be increased, not only to help in the fight against heart disease but also against breast and colon cancer.

The role that diet plays in immunologic competence is extremely important and scientists are beginning to recognize that certain foods help to maintain a healthy immune system. Foods that contain high levels of vitamins A, C, and E should be emphasized in our daily diet as a preventive measure.[7]

It's still unclear how human breast cancer starts. But it is on the upswing in this country and, therefore, every woman should get to know her breasts.

DESCRIPTION OF THE BREASTS

The breasts, or mammary glands, are made up of soft tissue and glands surrounded by fat. These glands are arranged in a complicated pattern of lobes not unlike the form of a wagon wheel. The milk ducts lead into the nipple. On the nipple, there are about 25 openings that connect to the ducts in an organized pattern. If a pregnancy occurs, the glands will produce milk for the baby's nutrition. Around the areola (the circular area around the nipple) are little glands that enlarge during pregnancy that lubricate the nipple during nursing.

There are many factors that determine the size and shape of the breast, such as genetics, nutrition, pregnancy, and hormones. The glandular tissue in the breasts varies with the bodily level of estrogen during a woman's normal monthly cycle, causing the breasts to increase and decrease in size. Fatty tissue fills out the breasts, making them round and smooth. The breasts are supported by muscles against the chest wall and ligaments that attach to the ribs, shoulders, clavicle, and sternum.

Losing weight will often get rid of some of the fat and make the breasts smaller. Certain exercises, like aerobics, will develop muscles in the vicinity of the breasts, making them seem larger and firmer. Extremely large breasts or premature development of the breasts can be a sign of a disorder, possibly a glandular one. Breasts may be firm and high or flaccid and pendulous.

The shape of the breast appears in many cases to be inherited. The breasts change shape during pregnancy due to the increase of glandular tissue and the engorgement caused by the production of milk. At menopause, the breasts change shape due to the lack of hormonal stimulation from the ovaries. Women with large breasts sometimes have breast reductions done at this time for cosmetic reasons.

LYMPH NODE DRAINAGE FROM THE BREAST

It is very important for a surgeon or oncologist treating breast cancer and the patient to know the anatomy of the breast. They should know the blood supply coming into the tissue (arterial) and the blood supply draining the area (venous) and more important, know the lymph gland drainage of the breast.

The woman then will better understand the importance of checking certain body areas during a breast self-examination. One area to be checked is the glands under the armpit. The breast has many lymphatic channels that can carry cancer cells away from the breast tissue to the glands, and when they become involved a metastases, or spread, has developed and treatment methods change.

The distribution of the lymphatic drainage of the breast came to light through research started many years ago. Mercurial injection techniques

Figure 1
ANATOMY OF THE FEMALE BREAST—LYMPHATIC DRAINAGE

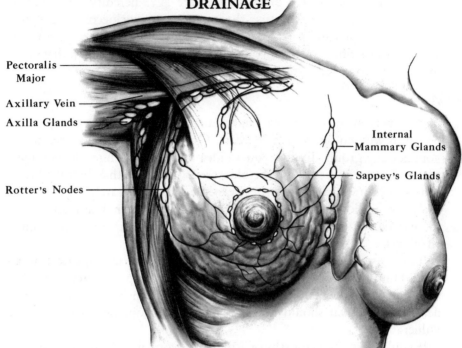

were used to evidence the many channels under the nipple. This, incidentally, is why tumors in this area can spread out in many different directions. The main lymphatic collecting channels lead to the axilla, or armpit.[8]

Another lymphatic drainage area passes beneath the chest wall muscles (pectoralis major muscles) and leads to the apex of the axilla (armpit). The lymph glands (nodes) between the pectoralis major and minor muscles are known as Rotter's nodes.[9]

What all this means is that the primary site of the breast tumor helps determine where the cancer will spread if it gets into the lymphatic channels. The main channels are the axilla (armpit) for lateral site tumors and the internal mammary chain (under the sternum) for medial site tumors. It is more difficult to determine where tumors under the nipple (subareolar) will spread (Sappey's nodes).[10]

Despite all we've learned about the anatomy of the human breast, it's still unclear as to how human breast cancer starts. It may begin when many risk factors join together to trigger the development of the disease.

IMPORTANT RISK FACTORS

The key risk factors for breast cancer are age, heredity, race, parity, weight, diet, hormonal status, thyroid disease, socioeconomic status, stress, drugs, precancerous mastopathy, previous cancer in one breast, or a cluster of calcification found on mammography. Admittedly, that's a lot of territory to cover. Let's review each factor separately.

Age

Ninety percent of the breast cancers that I have treated in my practice began in women older than 38 years. Only 10 percent developed in the younger age group. To give you an idea of the total range, the youngest patient I treated was 24 and the oldest was 95. More than half the breast cancers occurred in patients between the ages of 38 and 54 years. The majority developed breast cancer at menopause or later. This really serves to underscore the necessity of monthly self-examination and annual checkups.

It suggests that hormonal changes that occur at menopause play an important role in the etiology of breast cancer. As a patient gets older, her ability to charge up her immune system to fight cancer and other diseases decreases. Women should be aware that at menopause, they are more vulnerable.

If you're like three-fourths of American women, you found an excuse not to examine your breasts this month, either because you didn't know how, what to look for, or were afraid of what you'd find. Here is a chance to change that pattern: If you don't know how to examine your breasts, ask your doctor to show you how to do it properly. If you are in the higher risk group or over age 38, ask that a mammogram be done.

Heredity

In families where breast cancer strikes several members, questions about a genetic link become inevitable. In my practice, seven percent of patients with breast cancer had mothers with the disease and 21 percent had aunts, grandmothers, or sisters with breast cancer.

Heredity and genetic factors have been previously studied. Numerous researchers, including Dr. Abraham M. Lilienfeld[11] and Dr. Madge T. Macklin[12] showed there is a marked increase in breast cancer when female relatives have breast cancer, including cousins, aunts, and grandmothers. My own experiences with breast cancer patients substantiates these studies.

Figure 2
RISK FACTORS

RISK FACTORS	Breast Cancer Incidence*

Age

10%	50%	40%

Years   38   Menopause   54   90

← 90% after 38 yrs. of age →

Heredity	Family history of breast cancer Family history other types cancer
Race	Higher incidence among white women--world wide
Children	Nulliparous (no children) Late birth of first child
Menopause	Women who continue menstruating late in life-- over 50 yrs.
Weight	Overweight
Diet	High triglyceride diet (high in fat, low in fiber) High beef intake.*
Hormones	Early start of menstruating (before 12 yrs.) ? Birth control pill ? Estrogen therapy
Thyroid Problems	Usually hypothyroid. ? Stress
Socioeconomic status	Affluent, high income (may be related to diet)
Stress	? personality, depression
Drugs	Women exposed to DES
Precancerous mastopathy	Atypical hyperplasia, papillomatosis, etc.
Cancer in one breast	Second breast at greater risk
Suspicious mammograms	Clusters of calcifications, etc.

*Author's statistics

This means that if breast cancer is prevalent in your family, you are at greater risk for the disease, and you should see your doctor a little more often, be particular about your diet, exercise regularly, and have a screening mammogram earlier than the suggested time. Once you reach 38 years of age you should have an annual mammogram. You should also be diligent about doing breast self-examination. If you detect a lump or any other abnormality, consult your doctor. Please, don't postpone the visit.

Children (Parity)

Another important factor in breast cancer is whether the patient has had children, and how many. There is little question that nulliparous women (those who have no children) are high-risk candidates. It has also been widely accepted that bearing the first child at an early age confers some protection, for reasons yet unknown. In one study of Catholic nuns, Dr. J. F. Fraumeni[13] found the incidence of breast cancer dramatically higher than in the general female population. Other researchers[14] have shown that unmarried women have a higher risk of malignant tumors affecting the breast and reproductive organs.

Women who continue to menstruate late in life also have an increased risk for breast cancer. I carefully watch childless women and those who are still menstruating after age 50 and recommend more frequent examinations, including regular examination of the uterus and ovaries as well as the breasts.

Race

Not only does breast cancer seem to be centered geographically, it also has a higher incidence among white women than women of other races—a pattern that seems to prevail worldwide.

According to epidemiologists (those who study epidemic diseases including cancer in relation to environment and ways of life), the woman most likely to develop breast cancer is white, of northern European descent, overweight, had a relative with cancer, began menstruating early, and had her first child after she was 35 years old.

Still, the incidence of breast cancer continues to rise for both white and black females in this country, whereas in the Far East and Japan, the incidence of breast cancer is much lower.

Weight and Diet

Being overweight increases the risk of developing a malignant breast tumor. Excess weight can also make it more difficult to locate a tumor.

When my patients were asked whether they felt they were of average weight, below average, or overweight before they developed breast cancer, half said they were overweight and only a few said they were underweight.

When asked which specific foods were their dietary staples, 45 percent named steak and hamburgers. Cheese, butter, eggs, ice cream, and fried foods were also high on the list. All of this is further evidence that a diet high in animal fat and low in fiber is obviously linked with a tendency to develop breast cancer. This is discussed in more detail in Chapter 22, Cancer and the Foods You Eat.

Hormones and Menopause

Women who begin menstruating at an early age (in the United States, before 12) are more likely to develop breast cancer. On the other hand, if a woman has her ovaries removed before she is 35, or has a natural menopause at an early age, her chances of developing breast cancer drop considerably.

The female sex hormone, estrogen, has long been known to produce breast cancer in animal experiments[15] and has also been shown to cause precancerous changes in breast tissue in humans. The lining of the ductal system of the breast can be stimulated by hormones (estrogens) to cause a condition (hyperplasia) that is known to lead to breast cancer.

There is substantial evidence that indigenous hormones are involved in the causation of breast cancer—estrogens in particular. A study recently done in Sweden[16] suggests that the risk of breast cancer increases after perimenopausal treatment with estrogens and combinations of estrogen and progestin. It was originally thought that by adding progestins, the risk of getting endometrial cancer could be reduced, and that combination therapy might reduce any excess risk associated with long-term estrogen treatment.[17] But this and other studies suggest that routine use of estrogen-progestin drugs given at the menopause to prevent osteoporosis and other symptoms should be weighed carefully.

Estrogens are used in oral contraceptives and are also often used in the treatment of hot flashes during menopause. While some physicians feel that estrogens help prevent the crippling disease called osteoporosis, research has shown that women who have never taken estrogen suffer less often from malignant tumors.

When asked whether they took oral contraceptives or not, 15 percent of my patients who developed breast cancer said they had. Whether oral contraceptives actually cause cancer in humans is still a controversy.

Only further study will show if they produce carcinogenic effects on the breast, and if so, in what numbers. Fortunately, though, the oral contraceptives now in use have much lower estrogen contents than when they were first introduced over 30 years ago, and the risk factor may be lower.

Many women have their uterus and ovaries removed prior to menopause and, since ovaries are the major source of estrogens, replacement therapy is often given. Seventeen percent of the breast cancer patients I treated had a total hysterectomy (uterus) and bilateral oophorectomy (ovaries). Estrogen replacement therapy varied in dosage but all received it. From this, it's easy to see that when the ovaries are removed and replacement therapy is given, a woman can still get breast cancer and there is no protective effect from the removal of the ovaries.

If you need replacement estrogen therapy, the minimum dose should be used. If combination therapy is given it should be carefully adjusted by your physician.

More information on hormones and their relationship to breast cancer can be found in Chapter 8.

Thyroid

Researchers[18,19,20] have been working for years on the relationship between thyroid disease and breast cancer. They are certain there is a connection that involves iodine deficiency. However, it is difficult to establish the exact level of risk involved. Twenty percent of my breast cancer patients had a history of thyroid problems and seven percent had been operated on for thyroid disease. As for how the thyroid gland is involved in breast cancer, is not clear at the present time. Hypothyroidism seems to be a causative risk factor. The thyroid gland plays a role not only in maintaining a stable metabolism in the human body, but in stress and the immune system as well. If you have a breast problem and have thyroid disease you probably should be more alert to the signs of breast cancer.

Environment

Only within the past few years has much attention been paid to the environment in relation to breast cancer. Today, we have more and more potentially harmful substances all around us, and the "why" of breast cancer has become increasingly significant.

For example, women who live in cities have a higher incidence of breast cancer than those in rural areas. Those with higher incomes and higher social status are at greater risk[21]—presumably because they can afford the foods that compose a diet rich in fat and chemical additives. The water you drink, the food you eat, and the air you breathe have a definite effect on the cells of the human body. Be discerning of the water you drink. Read the labels on the food you buy. Try to avoid contaminated air. These basic steps are recommended not just to reduce the risk of breast cancer, but to promote wellness and well-being in general.

Stress

The relationship of stress and women's status in society might be called the social psychology of cancer. There is no longer any doubt that stress has a marked effect on the body's functions and plays a role in the etiology of cancer.

As for how the physician should evaluate stress as a risk factor in breast cancer, a few points can be made here. There is growing evidence that resistance to cancer is immunologic in nature, and that several stress factors are exhibited in many patients with cancer. They are: depression prior to cancer development, relative inability to express hostile feelings, unresolved tension concerning a familial figure, and sexual problems.

Among my breast cancer patients, nearly 40 percent said they had been under severe stress before their breast cancer was discovered. In contrast, among noncancerous control patients, a similar personality pattern involving stress was found in only 10 percent.

Smoking

Women who smoke may not necessarily develop breast cancer, but they are at higher risk for lung cancer, stomach ulcers, and heart disease.[22] The lung is also a common site for spread of breast cancer, and the damaging effects of smoking complicate the role of the physician. If my patient has breast cancer and smokes, she is vigorously advised to quit. Any way is o.k.—cold turkey, clinics, hypnosis—just as long as she quits. Not only does it make the patient feel better, and more empowered to control her body, it makes my job easier, too.

Previous Breast Lumps and Surgical Biopsy as Risk Factors

Before the development of newer diagnostic aids to help the surgeon determine which patients needed to be biopsied for possible breast cancer, many women in the 1960's and early 1970's had biopsies whenever they developed a new breast lump. The most common reason for biopsy was fibrocystic disease and there were many surgeons who felt fibrocystic disease was a precancerous condition.

Caffeine, chocolate, tea, and certain other foods have been suggested as causative factors in fibrocystic disease. Biopsies of numerous patients with fibrocystic disease have allowed for a study of such patients who have been watched for many years since their tissue diagnosis. I reviewed all my patients who were biopsied with a tissue diagnosis of fibrocystic disease (more than 500 cases studied for 25 years): less than one percent went on to develop cancer of the breast. It is my belief, therefore, that fibrocystic disease is not a precancerous condition.

Precancerous Mastopathy

Changes within the ductal system of the breast; hyperplasia, atypical hyperplasia, and some in situ carcinomas are difficult to differentiate from cancers in the development stage. Many physicians consider lobular carcinoma in situ (LCIS) to be more a marker of hyperplastic breast epithelium than a true malignancy. Diffuse intraductal papillomas in the breast are also considered premalignant lesions and these patients have to be examined and tested by mammograms more often.

Previous Cancer in One Breast

If a patient has a cancer in one breast the chances of her developing cancer in the second breast increase 3 to 7 percent. Unfortunately, much of the research on the bilaterality of breast cancer was done prior to the increased use of mammography and is not up to date. Today, an increasing number of synchronous (bilateral) breast cancers are being detected by mammography.[23]

As more minimal cancers are being detected, breast conservation treatment (lumpectomy and axillary dissection) is becoming more common. Most of these patients receive radiation treatments to the breast after a lumpectomy. However, exposure to ionizing radiation is considered to be a risk factor for breast cancer. This means that the second breast is at risk because radiation has a tendency to affect the opposite breast. Sarcomas (another form of cancer) can also develop in regions of the breast and chest wall where high doses of radiation are applied.

A group of cancer specialists in France[24] recently attempted to evaluate the incidence of second cancers in patients undergoing breast conservation followed by mega-voltage x-ray therapy. The study consisted of 2,850 patients with operable breast cancer (Stage I-III). Six and one-half percent of the patients developed a contralateral breast cancer. The future outlook for these patients who had cancers develop in both breasts was clearly less favorable than those patients who had cancer in only one breast—fifteen-year survival of 42 percent and 65.5 percent, respectively. See chapter 16 that discusses the care and management of the second breast.

Suspicious Mammographic Findings

The number of cancers of the breast detected by mammography continues to increase. As x-ray machines improve and the personnel reading the films gain more experience, the accuracy increases. While this diagnostic procedure is not perfect, mammography is still the only imaging device that can detect nonpalpable breast cancers two to four years before they can be felt.

In a study done on my breast patients, the accuracy of detecting breast cancers by mammography was 90 percent. This means the other 10 percent were detected by other means. Breast self-examination and careful examinations by health professionals are still necessary. Sometimes ultrasound testing or needle biopsy of difficult mammographic cases has to be done for early detection. Clusters of calcifications seen on mammography are particularly dangerous and in most cases should be biopsied.

SUMMARY

In considering risk factors, there are subtle but important distinctions to remember. Risk factors may not be actual cause and effect. For example, living in a city may be coincidental, not contributory—no one knows. Yet a woman must consider the high-risk factors that have been identified. She should also be sure her physician is aware of her risk status, for as a woman approaches menopause her jeopardy increases and continues to rise for the rest of her life. And although these are medical facts, each woman is a separate individual and her own risk factors may vary widely from those of other women. If you are in a high-risk group, you should see your doctor frequently. Remember: The risks outlined here are real, but they are also manageable.

2

Breast Self-Examination

The early detection of breast cancer is extremely important for this simple reason: if a breast cancer is detected when it is small there is less chance that it has spread; treatment methods, therefore, are more conservative and cure rates much better.

Today, there are three main diagnostic modalities for early detection: monthly breast self-examination, a thorough breast examination by a physician, and the use of diagnostic and screening mammography.

Until recently most lumps were first detected by the patient, who in turn often consulted the obstetrician, gynecologist, or surgeon. It was not until the early 1960's that x-ray techniques (mammography) were used to penetrate the breast tissue, detecting abnormalities and lesions that could be harbingers of cancer. The technique has been perfected and over 90 percent of breast cancers can be diagnosed in this way.

Sometimes ultrasound is used to determine if a lump is solid or cystic. This has been helpful in avoiding unnecessary biopsies. Despite the use of all methods of early detection there is still a 10 percent error rate in early diagnosis. Usually mammograms or ultrasound are done on an annual basis, and lumps can grow between examinations and can be detected by the patient. Twenty percent of my patients detected their breast cancers between their annual mammograms and thereby helped themselves to an earlier diagnosis and more effective, expedient treatment.

Breast self-examination can save your life. Detecting breast cancer early, when the disease is in a more curable stage, allows for many new options in treatment and increases the chance of successful medical care.

Women know they should examine their breasts, but most don't. Approximately 27 percent of American women examine their breasts on a monthly basis, leaving a 3-to-1 majority out of touch with signals their bodies may be sending.

When women in screening programs are taught to examine their breasts, more of them will detect their own cancers. So why don't more women examine their breasts? One reason is that they haven't been taught to understand just what they're feeling. Breasts are naturally somewhat lumpy. Breasts contain glandular tissue, fat, connective tissue, and lie over bone. Women aren't sure what's normal because they have never had a doctor or nurse take their hand, put it over their breast and say, "Feel this—this is your rib, this is a gland, this is breast tissue." Most women have to be taught how to do a comprehensive breast self-examination.

Some women refuse to do breast self-examination because they are apprehensive and fearful that they will misinterpret what they feel. If this is the case, they should ask their doctor or nurse to do it for them, or at least show them how (see Figure 3). Since most lumps are benign, many fears can be allayed with one easy visit to the doctor.

Until mammography was introduced, the only method of detecting cancer was by feel (palpation). Women would often rush to their doctor whenever a hard area developed in their breast. Many unnecessary biopsies were performed; as many as 10 to 15 biopsies would be done to detect one breast cancer. With the introduction of needle biopsy and mammography, most unnecessary surgery is now avoided. In my practice today (1991) one out of four biopsies is positive.

Who should a woman consult if she feels a lump in her breast? An obstetrician is a good choice. In fact, my survey of breast cancer patients revealed obstetricians as the most frequently consulted physician (12 percent).

Many hospitals provide individual instruction in breast self-examination (BSE) as part of their screening and diagnostic services. The American Cancer Society's Teach-In Program gives free group instruction through local chapters. Instruction is given in the American Cancer Society booklet, also available from local chapters. Many hospitals and local medical societies also have breast detection programs.

Some instructions on BSE, though excellent, may omit some warning signs. This chapter will try to explain a method that works. If you have any further questions, you should consult your physician.

ONCE A MONTH, EVERY MONTH

Women over 20 years of age should examine their breasts once a month, every month. It should be made part of a monthly routine. The best time for examination is right after your menstrual period, so that you can become familiar with the way your breasts normally feel.

If you are in the age group for which annual mammograms are recommended, you should still do monthly breast self-examinations. If you notice a change that persists through the menstrual cycle—a lump, swelling, or other symptom—you should see a doctor right away. Never try to diagnose yourself.

Fortunately, most lumps prove to be benign, but (see Chapter 7, Breast Lumps That Are Not Cancer) some characteristics suggest cancer more strongly than others. For example, a lump that feels stony, rigid, or has uneven edges should alert a woman to call her doctor. Skin dimpling, inversion of the nipple, or a bloody nipple discharge should also be investigated.

Women who have had a hysterectomy (removal of the uterus) but whose ovaries are intact may be able to tell when they are ovulating and should mark that date as a time for doing breast self-examination. Ovulation usually occurs in the middle of the menstrual cycle and may be accompanied by pain or discomfort in the lower abdomen. If a woman has had her ovaries removed she should select a specific day of the month for examining her breasts and continue the routine for the rest of her life.

Because breast cancers can still be found by women who have had regular mammograms, all women should perform monthly breast self-examination, paying special attention to the upper outer quadrant of the breast and armpit area, where a high percentage of cancers appear (see Figure 4). Breast self-examination can be done in many different ways, and one method may be better than another. But the importance of BSE increases as a woman gets older, and the monthly exam teaches a woman where small abnormalities are, so a new lump can be easily recognized.

Figure 3
BREAST SELF-EXAMINATION (BSE)

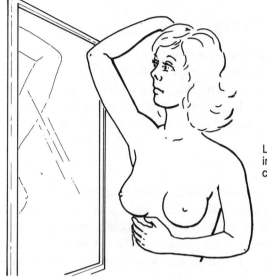

Look for skin
indentation, size
change and asymetry.

MIRROR INSPECTION

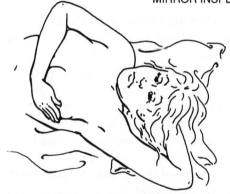

Feel for lumps completely
around the breast. Check
armpit. Press firmly, then gently.

LYING DOWN--PALPATING BREASTS

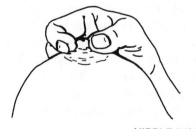

Squeeze nipple for
discharge: ? Bloody.
? Ulceration or other
abnormalities.

NIPPLE INSPECTION

The method of examination the patient feels most comfortable with is the one she should use.

HOW IT SHOULD BE DONE

There are several ways to examine your breasts, but a three-stage procedure is the most effective: mirror inspection, breast palpation, and soaping the breasts. This is easy to do and can save your life, but remember, no single method of breast examination is completely guaranteed to evidence the many symptoms of breast cancer. If you have any doubts, see your doctor.

Mirror Inspection

Stand in front of a large mirror and examine your breasts visually—first with your arms hanging at your sides, then with your hands pressing inward and down on your hips to contract the pectoral muscles (underneath your breasts). Next, press your palms together at heart level and, finally, clasp your hands behind your head. Here are some of the things you should be looking for:

1. *Skin dimpling.* If the previously round contour of the breast becomes concave at any point, showing a dimple, the depression may indicate the pull of a tumor.
2. *Inversion of the nipple.* A nipple that changes direction—pointing inward instead of projecting, or markedly shifting its angle—may signal an embedded tumor. It can also be the result of fibrocystic disease, calcium deposits, or previous surgery.
3. *Sore or irritated nipple.* One type of breast cancer is associated with nipple changes—Paget's Disease of the nipple. Usually in this affliction the nipple becomes reddened. It also may become thickened and hard, or there may be a sore-like ulceration or erosion. When the nipple develops a sore like this your doctor should be consulted and a biopsy (removal of a piece of the nipple tissue) should be done so the tissue can be studied in the lab.
4. *Nipple discharge.* Relax: only 5 percent of nipple discharges (bloody) are associated with cancer. Most bloody nipple discharges are usually discovered by the patient. The color can be red, green, or black, and might be noticed on the bed or underclothing. The discharge is usually due to small growths within the ductal system of the breast that erode small blood

Figure 4

LOCATION OF MOST BREAST CANCER LUMPS

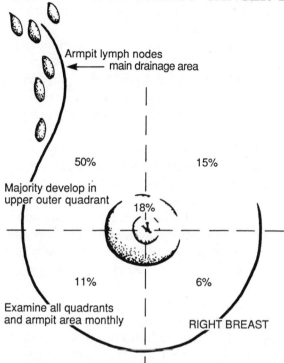

Armpit lymph nodes
←——— main drainage area

50%

15%

Majority develop in
upper outer quadrant

18%

11%

6%

Examine all quadrants
and armpit area monthly

RIGHT BREAST

Statistics Source: National Cancer Institute

vessels. You should see your doctor if this occurs. A clear yellow or white discharge from the breast is quite common and is almost always benign. It should not be confused with a bloody discharge. See Chapter 3 for a more thorough discussion of nipple discharge.

5. *Redness of the skin or blotching.* A rare form of cancer, inflammatory carcinoma, can cause the breast skin to redden or become blotched as it would from infection or irritation. This is due to the rapid growth of blood vessels within the tumor, which discolors the skin surface. If this condition persists it requires a biopsy for accurate diagnosis. The biopsy should include skin.

6. *Breast size.* Compare your two breasts. If a breast suddenly increases in size it may mean a cyst has formed and filled with fluid or a solid growth may have finally become noticeable. If this is confirmed by "feel," your doctor should be consulted. Many rapid increases in the size of a breast are attributed to cysts that

often can be aspirated by your doctor and may not require surgery. If the breast has gotten smaller on one side, it may be due to puckering of the breast tissue by a growth in the deeper part of the breast. This too should be investigated.

7. *Armpit lump.* The armpit (axilla) is a common site for a lump that may be indicative of a tumor. This is where breast cancer cells frequently drain to and is where the spread of breast cancer often occurs. In fact, a woman can have a large lump under her armpit and not be able to feel any irregularity in the breast tissue itself. In other words, one can have a very tiny cancer in the breast, not be able to feel it, and the first symptom that develops is a lump under the armpit. When this occurs, the doctor should be consulted and frequently a diagnostic workup, including a mammogram, must be done.

8. *Orange peel skin (peau-d'orange).* A peculiar orange-peel appearance to the skin of the breast sometimes develops. This unusual enlargement of the pores and roughness of the skin texture can be caused by a tumor that blocks channels carrying lymph fluid to and from the breast.

9. *Breast injury.* Any injury to the breast can cause blood to accumulate under the skin (hematoma) or scarring and destruction of fatty tissue. This can result in a lump or swelling that may be confused with cancer. It can also cause difficulty interpreting an x-ray (mammogram). If the lump persists an aspiration biopsy should be done.

10. *Areola.* Any noticeable variation of the dark halo or areola that surrounds the nipple, such as puckering or swelling, is a warning signal. It should be checked by a physician.

Breast Palpation

In this technique, the woman lies down, places a small pillow or towel under her shoulder on the side of the breast to be examined, then raises that arm above her head. What this does is to bring the breast tissue up on the chest wall so that the undersurface of the breast can be examined better (particularly helpful for large-breasted women). It affords a different approach to feeling the breast than in the sitting or standing position. However, in the sitting position, when some women lean forward, they can feel the contents of their breasts better than in the supine, or lying down, position.

The palm of the opposite hand, with the fingers closed, is used in palpating the breast. Visualize a clock with the upper portion of the breast at 12 o'clock and the lower portion at 6 o'clock. Next, examine the armpit by squeezing the fingers under the muscle and feeling for lumps. Then use the palm of the hand to firmly compress the breast tissue against the chest wall. At the lower curve of the breast, there is a normal ridge of firm tissue. Repeat the exam in a clockwise fashion but do not compress the tissue as firmly. This allows you to feel smaller, more subtle changes. Lastly, the nipple and subareolar tissue (under the nipple of the breast) is gently squeezed between the thumb and forefinger to see if there is any abnormal or bloody discharge from the nipple. The opposite breast is examined in the same manner.

The following abnormalities are what you should be looking for.

1. *Internal lumps.* Most breast lumps are harmless. New lumps, particularly if hard or fixed, or old ones that have grown, may indicate a tumor.
2. *Thickened tissue.* Bands of thick, fibrous tissue that can be felt in the upper parts of heavy breasts and in the "shelving margin" underneath the breast are a concern if they suddenly change in size.
3. *Breast contour.* Any change in the contour or shape of the breast can be a warning sign as can puckering, swelling, or dimpling.
4. *Nipple changes.* Look for scaling, inversion, or discharge, either bloody or clear.
5. *Armpit lumps.* Often overlooked, the axilla (armpit) must also be palpated for growths. Bear in mind that the quarter of the breast closest to the armpit is the site of about half of all breast cancers.

Soaping the Breasts

Many of my patients tell me they first found a lump while taking a bath or shower. This is not surprising, since bumps and dips in breast tissue feel like mountains and valleys beneath fingertips slick from soap or bath oil. Of course, you are still looking for any of the symptoms already discussed. Whether you use soap to improve the tactile feel of your examination is up to you.

WHEN ONE SHOULD NOT DO BREAST SELF-EXAMINATION

Some women are so nervous about their breasts that breast self-examination creates more problems than it's worth. Because of the publicity concerning cancer and the heightened fear of cancer of the breast, some women cannot examine their breasts without becoming terrified and emotionally drained. These individuals would be better off letting their doctors examine their breasts periodically.

WHAT IF YOU FIND A LUMP?

If you find something new during your breast self-examination, don't panic. Swelling rarely indicates the growth of new tissue, and even more rarely is it cancerous. Again, remember: most breast lumps are benign. If you have any doubts, most communities have specialists in the diagnosis and treatment of cancer. They can be found in the telephone directory under oncology or oncologists, or you can check with your local medical society for the names of cancer specialists near you. The Cancer Information Service of the National Cancer Institute has a toll-free number (800-638-6694) for current information on cancer specialists and hospitals, as do other organizations (see Appendix B).

If you have reservations concerning diagnosis and treatment, you should seek a second opinion from a physician or surgeon of your choosing—not someone recommended by the first doctor. The "buddy system" among doctors may prevent you from getting an unbiased opinion. Sometimes, going outside the local community for a second opinion is advised to ensure an impartial consultation.

In some cases, the diagnosis and treatment may be so difficult to determine that a medical consensus is necessary. This has led to Tumor Boards in large community hospitals, where many specialists combine to share their knowledge and opinions to help the breast cancer patient. A Tumor Board, however, is only as good as the people who serve on it.[25] The Board should be comprised of doctors who are true cancer specialists representing all the major disciplines that serve cancer patients. The members should include medical oncologists, surgical oncologists, radiation therapists, pathologists, and immunologists.

Steady strides continue to be made against breast cancer and cancers of

Figure 5
BREAST TUMOR SIZE AND DETECTION

Size of tumor seen on mammography
but cannot be felt

5 mm

Size of tumor first felt by
breast self-examination

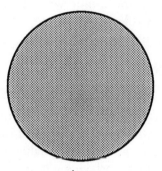

1 cm

Largest size of tumor
recommended for lumpectomy
(RX, controversial)

4 cm

If the tumor is this size
or larger, 50% will have
spread to other areas of
the body (metastases)

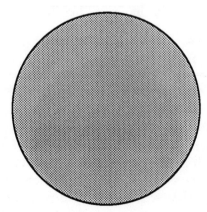

5 cm or larger

ACTUAL TUMOR SIZE

all types. Today, according to the American Cancer Society, there are over one-half million women who have survived breast cancer.

Survival rates have increased in recent years as a direct result of breast self-examination and mammography. It's becoming evident to everyone that breast cancer is often curable if diagnosed *and* treated early (see Figure 5).

This last dictum can't be overstressed. Among the patients in my survey, only half said they visited a doctor within one week of discovering a lump. Twenty percent waited three months or longer, and some took six months to a year before seeking any medical advice. It came as no surprise that in many of these patients who delayed their treatment, the cancer had spread outside the breast. In some cases the cancer, left unchecked, had pervaded the body.

The smaller the tumor when detected, the more breast care options there are available to the patient.

SUMMARY

Breast self-examination is a tried and true method of detecting breast cancer. Unfortunately, not all communities have cancer specialists, sophisticated x-ray machines, or ultrasound equipment—you may have to travel to find good cancer specialists and equipment. Remember, patients who find and report changes in their breasts between annual exams contribute greatly to their well-being. Monthly breast self-examinations should be done once a woman reaches her twentieth birthday and should be continued for the rest of her life.

QUESTIONS

Q. Should a woman still do breast self-examinations now that we have mammography?

A. Of course. Screening mammography is still not done on the majority of women, so many cancers can still be found by breast self-examination. Although mammograms are very useful, they are not perfect. When a woman stays "in touch" with her breasts, she is able to detect changes that occur between annual mammogram exams.

Q. How much do mammograms cost?

A. The price varies according to the community and the facilities that are used. A mammogram done in a mobile unit might cost $50, but the price can be as high as $200 elsewhere.

Q. *Why doesn't the government pay for mammograms if they're so good?*

A. The cost could be overwhelming since there are so many women who qualify.

Q. *Does the government pay for mammograms for Medicare patients, since breast cancer is prevalent in that age group?*

A. Yes. It does cover the charge for yearly mammograms.

Q. *Is it easy to learn how to do breast self-examination?*

A. Yes. Once you learn how to do it, you'll be able to detect small abnormalities in your breast better than women who are untrained in self-examination.

Q. *Are there some breasts in which it's more difficult to detect tumors?*

A. Yes. Bilateral hard, dense breasts are extremely difficult to examine. If there is diffuse fibrocystic disease present, sometimes it's almost impossible to detect a new lump.

Q. *What should a woman do if she has dense breasts that are difficult to examine?*

A. She will have to have mammograms done more often to detect early cancers, particularly if she is in a high-risk group. Breast self-examination is less effective in detecting some tumors, especially in dense breasts.

3

Nipple Discharge

A nipple discharge can be frightening, particularly if there is some blood in it. Fortunately, this is not a frequent sign of breast cancer. But it does scare the patient, however, and gets her into the doctor's office promptly. "I had some bright red blood on my bra," or "I have a greenish and yellowish discharge from my nipple," are typical of the reports made to the doctor.

If a discharge occurs before the age of 50, it's often a benign condition. If it develops after 50 years of age it has a stronger association with cancer. In the younger age group it's seen with the postpartum state, accompanying pregnancy, hormonal therapy, and certain drugs (such as chlorpromazine). It can also be associated with the use of birth control pills and some small tumors at the base of the brain (pituitary tumors) that secrete prolactin, a hormone that increases during pregnancy and is necessary for the growth and development of the breast in preparation for breastfeeding.

Usually if a discharge occurs from both nipples it's due to diffuse changes in the breasts and the discharge can be clear or milky. A nonspontaneous discharge from multiple ducts of both breasts is often due to diffuse symptomatic fibrocystic disease.

26

If a patient has a unilateral nipple discharge a cancer has to be excluded. However, the majority of these patients will still have a benign condition. Blood can be present in both benign and malignant conditions, so it cannot be stated that blood from the nipple is always associated with a malignant condition.

HOW A PATIENT WITH A NIPPLE DISCHARGE IS EVALUATED

First, a complete physical examination and review of the patient's medical history should be done. The color and amount of the discharge should be determined, as well as the time of the onset. Is the discharge bilateral or unilateral? Has the patient just had a pregnancy? Can the patient produce a discharge by squeezing the breast?

Usually the doctor will take sterile gauze and gently rub the nipple to eliminate any stoppage that may be preventing the discharge. He will then gently compress the nipple clockwise in all four quadrants to try to determine the duct or ducts responsible for the discharge. The discharge might be milky, red, green, watery and yellowish, purulent or sticky. Blood is easily recognized but if there is doubt, Hemostix or Wrights stain (microscopic slides) can be used to determine if blood or purulent cells are present.

A few years ago, I tried to correlate bloody discharge cases with cancer but found the cytological examination of the nipple discharge wasn't very helpful. The accuracy of the diagnosis was dependent on whether a fresh smear was taken, and whether the pathologist was accurate in determining the diagnosis by looking at the cells under the microscope. There were too many false-negative and false-positive findings to rely on the examination for a definitive diagnosis. Today, cytology has improved and can be helpful in difficult cases where the surgeon is undecided as to whether a biopsy should be done.

Mammography is sometimes helpful in defining breast changes responsible for nipple discharge—usually these are seen in larger, diffuse breast lesions and a tumor can be palpated. Small intraductal papillomas (little tumors inside the ducts) are difficult to identify even if the duct is cannulated by the surgeon prior to surgery. When more than one duct is involved with a papilloma, or if diffuse papillomatosis is present, careful microscopic examination has to be done to rule out cancer. This type of patient has to be followed more closely.

Magnification of mammograms can also be done to get a better look at the suspicious area. In some cases, injection techniques (galactography) into the ducts has helped identify the condition. Galactography takes time and is not available in all medical centers.

If a single duct discharge (bloody) persists intermittently and the mammogram remains normal, the duct system of the quadrant involved should be excised. This can be done by cannulating the duct and then excising the breast tissue from the nipple to the breast parenchyma. If the major duct system has to be excised and the patient is young, it means the patient would not be able to nurse an infant from that breast.

When the ductal system is excised, immediate frozen section diagnosis of the tissue is usually not helpful. Multiple tissue slices have to be made to detect small papillomas or small cancers, and many slides have to be examined to detect the small tumor.

SUMMARY

Fewer than 5 percent of the patients seen in my office during the past ten years who complained of a nipple discharge actually required surgery. Usually nipple discharges that are linked to cancer have a palpable mass, and only a small percentage of those cases fail to show some mammographic abnormality. When cancer is present but is not felt, it is almost always papillary, intraductal carcinoma in situ, or lobular carcinoma in situ and limited surgery can be done.

QUESTIONS

Q. *If a woman has a nipple discharge, how can she tell if blood is present?*

A. The color is usually brownish, bright red, or a greenish-brown color. The skin surface is acidic and the acid can cause a greenish discoloration to the blood. Hemostix available in drug stores can be used for complete accuracy.

Q. *What's the most common diagnosis when bright red blood is found?*

A. Intraductal papilloma, which is usually benign. Only about 5 percent of such cases are malignant.

Q. *Can the birth control pill cause a nipple discharge?*

A. Yes. This is usually clear and watery in consistency.

Q. Can Paget's Disease of the nipple have a bloody discharge?

A. Yes, although it is usually accompanied by an erosion of the nipple surface. All these lesions should be biopsied.

Q. Do young girls ever have a bloody nipple discharge?

A. They can. This can be associated with the onset of menses.

Q. Why do pregnant women get bloody nipple discharges?

A. The breasts sometimes get markedly engorged during pregnancy and small blood vessels can break.

Q. Can you get a bloody nipple discharge if you have inverted nipples?

A. Yes. Also seen are skin rashes like eczema of the skin of the breast, if it involves the nipple. Herpes simplex, abscesses, and small fistulas of the ducts can also cause a bloody nipple discharge.

Q. Does jogging cause a bloody nipple discharge?

A. It can. Traumatic erosion from the bra rubbing against the nipple can cause bleeding.

Q. When might a bloody nipple discharge require surgery?

A. When it's accompanied by a lump, when only one breast is involved, when it's from a single duct, when the mammogram is suspicious, or if the patient is over 45 years of age.

4

The Medical Examination You Can Expect

The medical examination you get is only as good as the physician who does it. It takes time to assess a woman's history and perform a competent physical examination and there is an art to doing it properly. Your doctor's training background is important when it comes to caring for a potential cancer patient. Is your doctor a specialist? Does he have his "boards" (or certification examination) in his specialty? Has he had specialized training at a cancer center? Does he do research in his area of expertise? If you're not sure of your doctor's credentials, you can contact the medical society in your community and they should give you the background of your doctor's training. If you have any doubts, don't hesitate to dig deeper for a second opinion. Beware of the doctor who is very gentle, pats your hand, and tells you everything is going to be all right.

By the time you reach menopause you should be having annual physical examinations. Many times these are done by the obstetrician who delivered your children or by an internist.

Two of the major diseases that plague women are highly curable if caught early: cancer of the breast and cancer of the cervix. Annual checkups can detect these cancers before they do serious harm. But more than half of all women fail to have complete physical examinations that include pap smears and the examination of the pelvic organs. A complete examination of the breasts, including a mammogram, should also be done.

The reasons women cite for not having an annual examination are: they can't be bothered to take the time, they're afraid of what might be found, or they can't afford it.

If you are in this blind majority it's important that you see a doctor once a year from now on, particularly if you're over 40. If you're younger and have experienced changes in your breasts that are disturbing to you or your doctor, you should have a baseline mammogram. This will provide a reference in case you develop a problem in the future. You should also tell the radiologist that you want the mammogram films saved for future comparison. If they are unwilling to save the films, request that they be given to you, since you paid for them. No one can deny you this information. It's your life you are trying to preserve.

A good checkup for cancer requires a complete patient history and a thorough physical examination. Your doctor should interview you to get a comprehensive history and determine whether you are in a high-risk group (See Chapter 1), and if a more extensive evaluation is needed. As previously mentioned, high-risk women are those who are over 35 years old: have a family history of breast cancer, have no children or had children late in life, began menstruating at an early age, are of northern European ancestry, or overweight.

The history your physician develops should also include previous surgery (especially for other cancers or any thyroid problems), whether you have taken hormone preparations for menopausal symptoms or birth control pills, and any other types of medications you may be taking, as some can alter the structure or appearance of breast tissue. Biopsy results of previous surgery should also be added to your medical history, as should any past mammograms.

The physical examination should include the skin, breasts, and organs of the chest, abdomen, and reproductive system. A vaginal examination is also essential. Allowing modesty to interfere with gaining a clear view of your health is, I believe, a reckless gamble. Also included in the exam should be a blood pressure check, electrocardiogram, height and weight, urinalysis, and a complete blood count, including cholesterol levels. Don't be alarmed if the doctor suggests other tests in addition to these. He may feel that it's wise to take all precautions.

If you have rectal bleeding, the doctor may suggest a proctosigmoido-scopy, colonoscopy, or barium enema. If there is any question about what is felt on pelvic examination, an ultrasound of the pelvic organs may be called for. Many new sophisticated tests such as CT scans (computerized tomography) and MRI scans (magnetic resonance imaging) are now available to aid both doctor and patient in securing an accurate diagnosis.

Palpation

Once the doctor has taken a complete history, your breasts will be examined using a method similar to that for breast self-examination. The patient disrobes and is first examined in the sitting position for any skin changes or bulges, nipple irregularities or discharge, and any difference in the size of the breasts. My experience has been that some breast conditions (bulges or dimples, in particular) can be more readily seen in a patient sitting or standing, as opposed to one who is lying down.

Next, the patient is told to lie down and the breasts are palpated for evidence of internal lumps or growths. The patient should not tell the doctor if or where she felt a lump so the physician will not be prejudiced. If the physician cannot find the lump, however, she should show him where she felt the change. The examination should also include palpation of the lymph glands in the adjacent armpits to detect if they are enlarged.

A stethoscope examination of the chest is then done to determine if the patient has any heart or lung problems. The abdomen is palpated and examined to see if the liver is abnormal (enlarged or nodular). The reason for this part of the examination is that estrogens, which have a lot to do with breast development, are detoxified in the liver and any damage to the liver from alcoholism may cause changes in the breast tissue. Meta-static cancer can also involve the liver.

Palpation, even by a doctor, can miss up to 20 percent of breast cancers. When used together with a biopsy, the figure drops precipitously.

Needle Aspiration

Needle aspiration is an inexpensive, cost-effective way of diagnosing breast tumors. In fact, it is the method of choice for many and eliminates the anxiety of waiting for a diagnosis. It can be done in the doctor's office under local anesthetic, avoiding the high cost of hospitalization.

However, needle aspiration can sometimes be difficult. If the patient has bilateral dense fibrotic breasts, where should the doctor insert the needle? If there are multiple nodules in both breasts it also creates a problem. Mam-mography may be helpful in this type of case but not always.

Needle aspiration of a suspicious lump in the breast has been used as a diagnostic tool for 65 years. In 1925, Dr. Hayes E. Martin[26] of New York's Memorial Hospital routinely aspirated all palpable tumors. Thirty years later, Dr. Otto Saphir[27] used needle aspiration on breast lesions occurring in pregnancy and lactation to diagnose breast cancer. Today, there is even less risk with the technique, and no evidence that tumor cells are disseminated by the procedure.[28,29] New methods of preparing and preserving the tissue sample for cytological diagnosis have also been vastly improved.

The only problem encountered is when needle aspiration is done by anyone other than a trained surgeon or radiologist, and is not done properly. The result can be hazardous, and sometimes lethal. The tumor can be missed and a false-negative result can occur. The needle has to be directed into the proper place and sufficient tissue removed for diagnostic purposes. It may be necessary to aspirate the suspected tumor in two or three different areas to obtain the proper sample. The recently developed multihole needle may solve this problem and appears to be less painful for the patient.[30] A Tru-cut needle can also be used.

If the breast exam reveals an obvious cyst (which is quite common), a needle aspiration can be done under local anesthetic in the doctor's office. If the aspirated fluid contains blood or cellular tissue it can be sent to a laboratory for analysis. The patient is then advised to return in one month to be sure the cyst has not refilled and that there is residual tissue present that may be a tumor. In rare cases, a cancer can be right next to a cyst or can grow within the tissue wall of the cyst and a biopsy is needed. The following case illustrates this point.

Fifteen years ago, I was asked to give a second opinion on a breast case operated on in a small hospital. The patient was a 34-year-old nurse who had a persistent lump. Two needle aspirations revealed the presence of a clear, yellow fluid. She decided that she wanted to have the lump removed. The surgeon removed the lump, which turned out to be a cyst. When the final tissue analysis was completed, it showed a small cancer in the lining of the cyst. Her surgeon told her the cancer was out and to forget about it. She went to New York and was advised to have a modified radical mastectomy and axillary dissection. I reviewed the first surgeon's operative report. In it, he described that the cyst had ruptured during the operative procedure.

I felt there were still cancer cells present in that breast and a further operation should be done. Breast conservation procedures were not popular yet, so a modified mastectomy was advised. As it turned out, the breast specimen showed an infiltrating ductal cancer at the site of the previous operation. Surgery was successful, the patient has since had a reconstruction of her breast (silicone implant), and she is alive and well.

Not all breast cancers can be diagnosed by needle aspiration, however, and cytological examination can occasionally provide false-positive results.[31] Examples of difficult diagnoses are: scirrhous carcinomas (stony tumors of the breast) and benign fibroadenomas or atypical histiocytes (scavenger cells present in connective tissue and lymph fluid). Inflammation and radiation effects on cell tissues can also make diagnosis more difficult. If there is any doubt, needle aspiration should be followed by an open biopsy of the suspected tumor.

Open Biopsy

In some large hospitals and cancer centers, needle aspiration is done more often than conventional open biopsy. However, my feeling is that this practice is not without risks. First of all, there is an inherent uncertainty in removing a breast (mastectomy) based solely on a small sample of tissue taken through a needle. If you're having an open biopsy or lumpectomy, there's no problem, since the diagnosis is confirmed and sufficient tissue is obtained for further study.

In small hospitals where aspiration techniques are limited and there are fewer cancer specialists, open biopsy should be done more often. In the past, a patient who went into a hospital for a breast biopsy often had her breast removed at the same time if the tissue sample proved malignant. This one-stage procedure is still the subject of great controversy and I believe should not be done. A two-stage treatment method should be used.

No woman should have to endure such a major procedure on such short notice, even if the biopsy immediately shows she has a malignant tumor. It's far better to schedule an operation *after* the biopsy has been confirmed and the physician can discuss the various treatment alternatives. This allows the patient's full participation in the treatment choice and means that she will be fully informed before giving her consent. It also allows her to get a second opinion if she doesn't trust the first doctor's judgment.

Mammography

Everyone is in agreement about the value of mammography (breast x-rays) in detecting tumors too small to be felt. What doctors disagree on is when the risks of radiation exposure—which in itself can cause breast cancer—outweigh the benefits. Fortunately, newer machines deliver small amounts of radiation to the breast—less than one rad per mammogram in most cases and as little as 3/10 rad in some larger hospitals that have the latest machines. With current low-dose equipment the risk of developing cancer from radiation exposure is minimal.

Who should have a mammogram and when should it be done on an annual basis? Sound clinical judgment is important in the evaluation of any breast cancer patient. No definite answers can be given, but I suggest the following guidelines:

1. Monthly breast self-examination after age 20. (I have had patients detect breast lumps at this age.)
2. Breast examination by a doctor once a year after age 38.
3. Mammogram, if necessary, in the young female if a lump is suspicious. (I have treated women with breast cancer as young as 24).
4. Screening mammogram at the age of 38 for a baseline study, and at an earlier age (35) if the woman falls into a high-risk group.
5. Mammograms every year after age 35, if the woman falls into a high-risk group. Routine mammogram on low-risk patients every two or three years.
6. More frequent and earlier mammograms if there is a strong family history of breast cancer and the suggestion of a genetic risk.

My own experience with mammography is that it should be done not only on women in the high-risk group, but on those who have large breasts or who are overweight. To explain this point, consider the case of a woman, 52, who was told by her doctor during a routine physical that she should have a mammogram. He said her breasts were so large that he couldn't tell by palpation if she had a tumor.

The mammogram showed a calcium deposit beneath the nipple, deep within the breast. However, there was no recognizable lump. As a precaution, a biopsy was then arranged. Microscopic examination of the tissue sample revealed a breast cancer. The patient was told the cancer was in an early stage and she elected to have a lumpectomy and axillary dissection. During the operation the lymph nodes in the armpit were examined and showed no evidence of spread of the tumor. This woman is alive today and her prognosis is excellent.

What Happens to My Tests? The importance of testing and analysis of breast cancer patients cannot be overemphasized. The American Cancer Society, in *Cancer Statistics*, reported in 1985 an 80 percent cure rate when breast cancer is detected early. Today the cure rate is approaching 90 percent. When the tumor has spread, not necessarily to distant sites, the figure drops to 60 percent. It also noted that only 52 percent of cases of breast cancer were detected at an early, localized stage. In other words, half of the women who develop breast cancer are not getting optimal treatment because the cancer is not detected early enough. Now that mammography is detecting minimal cancers, more tumors will be found at a localized stage.

The necessity for further tests should be decided on the basis of the patient's history or self-examination and the results of her physical examination by the doctor. Frequently the doctor will send you to a hospital, laboratory, or radiologist's office for the tests. Be sure you understand what the tests are, the specific instructions for taking them, and the results you can expect. Don't be afraid to ask questions.

To encourage hospitals to improve their anticancer efforts, the American College of Surgeons evaluates all hospital-based cancer programs. According to its *Cancer Program Manual*, the American Cancer Society is attempting to encourage each hospital or institution to improve its cancer-control efforts in the areas of prevention, early diagnosis, pretreatment evaluation, staging, optimal treatment, rehabilitation, and surveillance for recurrent and multiple primary cancers. For a current list of hospitals with approved cancer programs, you should contact the American Cancer Society (see Appendix B).

There's no doubt that cancer programs in some hospitals are better than others. The strength of a cancer program is dependent on the cancer specialists who work in the hospital and their training. Ask questions of all medical professionals who might assist you in evaluating the resources available to you.

Even though a doctor may be fairly certain a tumor exists from examination or x-rays, the tumor should be biopsied to determine whether it is benign or malignant. The tissue should then be examined under a microscope by a pathologist. He may also use special stains to determine the structure and activity of the individual cells to determine if they are cancerous and, if they are, what type. A portion of the tissue is analyzed for estrogen and progesterone to determine if the tumor is hormone-dependent. This information will be helpful in future treatment if the tumor spreads or metastasizes.

If the diagnosis of the tissue removed is questionable, then it can be sent to another pathologist at a different cancer center for analysis. For example, the Armed Forces Institute of Pathology in Washington, D.C., maintains a diagnostic center to aid hospitals in obtaining a proper tissue diagnosis, and to render second opinions for the patient. However, this is recommended only in the rare cases in which a diagnosis is in question.

SUMMARY

Scientists don't know why certain women get breast cancer and others don't. It is known that early detection reduces the chances that the cancer will spread, and that most cancer discovered early is curable. If you find a lump during breast self-examination, see a doctor at once. Rarely are such lumps malignant. If you have doubts about your doctor or your recommended treatment, remember you are dealing with your own body. There are enough good physicians available for you to be choosy.

Not every woman will examine her breasts. Not every woman who finds a lump will see a doctor. The fear of cancer distresses some women more than others. There's no reason to run away from the idea, however. Face it squarely, and you will see it's actually far less terrible than most people imagine. Cancer can be treated successfully and can be curable. We don't know all about it, but we do know a great deal.

QUESTIONS

Q. *Does it hurt to have a needle aspiration?*
A. Not very much. Still, the anxiety over having a needle stuck into the breast is too much for some women to bear, and a biopsy under general anesthesia may have to be considered.

Q. *Should you move directly from a biopsy to definitive surgery?*
A. No. The sample of tissue from the breast (biopsy) should always be thoroughly examined and this can take up to 72 hours, depending on the laboratory. This is more definitive than the "frozen section" technique used in one-stage mastectomy.

Q. *How does needle localization differ from aspiration?*
A. When a doctor does a needle localization, he uses a dye or hooked wire to pinpoint the growth in the breast before lumpectomy or other surgery. Most breast aspirations, on the other hand, are done to drain cysts or to make a preliminary diagnosis prior to major surgery. See Chapter 6, Needle Localization.

Q. Are some tumors harder to find than others?

A. Yes. Some breast tumors are not very cellular (atypical) and cytologists may miss the cancer or give a false-negative report. Scirrhous carcinoma of the breast is one such example of a difficult tumor to diagnose.

5

Imaging for Breast Tumors

Forty years ago, in order to detect a breast cancer, the patient or her doctor had to feel a lump. Fifty percent of breast tumors when first detected in the 1940's and 1950's showed evidence of spread (metastases) beyond the local area, indicating that very few women were alert to the problem. Even today, with information reaching hundreds of millions, only 30 percent of women do breast self-examinations.

In the past—as now—the emotional impact of detecting a lump sometimes led to withdrawal and denial, and a delay in seeking treatment. For some women with large or dense breasts, it was difficult to detect a tumor early. Pregnancy can also mask the signs of a hidden tumor.

The American Cancer Society—and the media—were instrumental in alerting the public to the value of breast self-examination. Pamphlets were distributed illustrating methods of examination, and physicians were advised to teach patients how to examine their breasts.

Unfortunately, in order to feel a new lump in a breast, the lesion has to be large enough to be detected by touch. This in itself means the lump has been growing in the breast for a while. With our modern knowledge of the growth of breast tumors, we know that it takes two to eight years to develop a malignancy of one centimeter (about the size of your thumbnail). This is the smallest size lump that can be felt in the breast.

A new method of early detection was needed so tiny tumors could be detected before they could be felt. Some way had to be found to penetrate and image the breast.

How does one image a gland, such as the breast, to detect changes without damaging the gland? After all, breasts differ widely in shape and size. Some youthful breasts are firm and uniformly hard. Aging causes glandular changes, which effect overall size. Pregnancy causes marked changes in breast parenchyma. Injury can occur and all kinds of hormonal factors, genetics, and nutrition play a role in how a woman's breasts develop and feel.

Fifty years ago, attempts were made to transilluminate the female breast employing a high-intensity light beam.[32] This technique, also called diaphanometry, involves shining a light through the breast to outline its interior. Different types of tissues transmit and scatter the light in distinct ways, enabling doctors to perceive abnormalities more clearly. The light used is infrared and its ability to pass through the tissues depends on the amount of fat, density of the skin, and amount of glandular structures in the breast.

Unfortunately, there was frequently a disparity between the x-ray findings and the optical findings. The one obvious advantage of transillumination is that it doesn't expose the breast to radiation. However, there were too many false-negatives and false-positives for practical screening purposes. Another method had to be found.

Injection techniques were also attempted. Radioactive chemicals were injected into the veins, hoping the chemicals would travel to the breast tumor site and could then be imaged. But there was little success with this technique.

Galactography is a method of taking x-ray pictures of the ducts that empty into the nipple by injecting a radiopaque contrast agent.[33] This is sometimes useful in the study of a nipple discharge—particularly if a bloody discharge from a single duct cannot be explained by a mammogram. However, its main use is in outlining the ducts and it has no real application for screening purposes.

Thermography was also tried.[34,35,36] Infrared photography was used to detect cancers by measuring the heat patterns emitted from the breasts. Cancerous areas are warmer than normal body tissues. This undertaking also had its drawbacks. Heat sensitivity is extremely difficult to calibrate. If the tumor is large, a large amount of heat is given off.

If the tumor is small, a small amount is registered, and the small tumors are difficult to detect. This is not exactly what the scientists were hoping for.

Thermography does have some useful application, however, in screening women who are not at risk. But the fact that false-positive results can lead to unnecessary biopsy generally rules out thermography as a viable means of early detection. Like transillumination, its limitations far outweigh the fact that the patient is not exposed to radiation.

Xeroradiography[40,41,42,43] The xerographic reproduction process was patented in 1942. In 1947, the Haloid Company (Xerox Corporation) began commercial development of the technology. Application to medicine began and xeroradiograms of the breast were first done in 1956. In this technique, the image of the breast is produced on a special coated paper, not on x-ray film. The use of xeroradiography has decreased because of the development and improvement of mammography with even lower radiation exposure.

In the 1970's, because of the fear of the potential carcinogenic effect of radiation (mammography) a renewed interest in ultrasound developed.[37,38,39] High-frequency sound waves are projected into the breast tissues to determine if a lump is solid (tumor) or cystic. Computers record the differences in densities of the breast tissues.

This technique is particularly helpful if the woman has large breasts or is apprehensive about needle aspiration. It's not as accurate as mammography, however, because of the difficulty in determining the differences between benign and malignant lesions. Today ultrasound is used to determine solid from cystic lesions in the breast, and is also used to examine other areas of the body, including the gallbladder, pancreas, kidneys, pelvis, uterus, and ovaries.

Mammography (x-ray imaging) is the method most frequently used in the 1990's to detect cancers of the breast. It was introduced in 1913 in Germany by a surgeon named Salomon.[44] At first, it was thought to be a primitive method, hazardous, and a curiosity, and didn't get medical support. In the 1930's, Stafford L. Warren,[45] a radiologist in Rochester, New York, reported on the clinical application of x-rays of the breast. New Eastman Kodak x-ray films were used and proper positioning of the patient for breast pictures was demonstrated. For a short time there was a renewed interest in using mammography but this quickly subsided.

Then, in the 1950's, a young radiologist, R. L. Egan, trained at the M. D. Anderson Hospital and Tumor Institute, investigated in depth the technique of mammography, and after studying dosimetry and quality of the x-ray beam, helped establish the mammography technique used today. In 1960 he published his experience with 1,000 cases.[46]

With the publication of his report, there was a renewed interest in mammography and Egan was named the principal investigator of a nationwide study: The M. D. Anderson Hospital, the Cancer Control Program (U.S.P.H.), the National Cancer Institute (N.C.I.) and 24 institutions scattered around the United States were designated to test the usefulness of mammography.

This combined study soon found that mammography x-ray is clearly the single most important modality in the early detection of breast tumors. Other important research studies were subsequently done.[47]

From 1963 to 1966, the Health Insurance Plan (H.I.P.) of New York conducted breast screening with a physical examination and Egan's technique of mammography to determine whether it could reduce breast-cancer mortality. Sixty thousand women were randomized in screening and control groups and it was found by the seventh year that the mortality in women 50 years of age and older was one-third lower in the screened than in the non-screened group. The value of mammography as a tool to detect small cancers of the breast was now quite evident.

In 1963, I began using mammography as a diagnostic tool with Dr. Paul Cooper, a radiologist at Hartford Hospital. At that time, we were criticized for exposing the breasts to excessive radiation. It was felt that ionizing radiation had clearly been shown to increase the risk of developing breast cancer.

As the radiologists became adept in detecting cancers, the interest in the technique by other doctors in our institution increased, and the value of mammography outweighed the risks. New x-ray machines were developed to decrease radiation exposure, and x-ray technicians were taught how to image the breast.

It soon became evident that imaging the breast is not an easy task. It's a difficult organ to image because of the effects of hormonal stimulation on the premenopausal breast. The geometry of the breast on the chest wall is complex and at times it can be difficult to get adequate views of the axilla. Very small, dense breasts, for example, are very difficult to image. Good mammography demands the highest sensitivity possible in order to image the fine structures and small calcification characteristics of early-stage breast cancer.

Excellent studies can only be done with a trained, coordinated team approach. Each individual involved has an important part to play—the machine performing the imaging cannot be useful unless its operators are astute in interpreting its data.

The x-ray technician is extremely important in positioning the breast prior to taking the picture. If the breast is positioned improperly, it means that more pictures have to be taken and there is more radiation exposure, hence more eventual breast-cancer risk for the patient. Vigorous compression of the breasts is necessary to avoid underexposing the base against the chest wall. The firmer the compression, the better the mammogram. This is why some women complain about the pain and discomfort associated with mammography. However, it is really a small price to pay for early detection—a few moments of discomfort for the awareness of the condition of your breasts.

A mammogram is also only as good as the radiologist who reads the films and interprets the picture. Your cancer surgeon should review the films as well. There is no doubt that specialists in radiology mammography are more accurate in interpreting mammographic films. A radiologist reading mammograms only occasionally will make mistakes.

If you have any doubts about your mammograms, get a second opinion from someone who reads mammograms every day.

CT Scan of the Breast (X-ray)

Computerized Axial Tomography of the body has become a major diagnostic tool in detecting abnormalities by cross-sectional images. A high-intensity x-ray beam is passed through the tissues to determine density and then a computer puts it on film for analysis.

Attempts to image the breast have also been tried by rotating a narrow x-ray beam around the breasts. This practice, unfortunately, exposes the breast to much more radiation than is normal during a mammogram and its disadvantages outweigh its advantages over mammography.

CT Scan Detection of Recurrent Disease

CT scans do have an important use in breast tumor detection of recurrent disease. The following case is a good illustration.

I was asked to see a 44-year-old white female who had had a right modified mastectomy four years earlier. She went to another surgeon because of severe right arm pain. Neurologists and neurosurgeons saw the patient in consultation and noted slight right arm nerve weakness but an explanation was not forthcoming. Her surgeon explored the chest wall area where the breast had been removed. The exploration was described essentially as negative for cancer.

I decided to do a CT scan of the chest wall. There was a suggestion of a cancerous mass at the thoracic outlet where the nerves go to the arm. I surgically removed this mass (which was, in fact, cancer) and the patient got prompt relief from her pain. Post-operative x-ray therapy and chemotherapy were given to ensure eradication of the cancer.

Magnetic Resonance Imaging[48,49,50]

The potential of this diagnostic device has only recently been recognized. In MRI, a large magnet—with a hole big enough for the patient to fit through—is surrounded by a radio-frequency transmitter. The images are produced on a computer printout, and can pinpoint tiny breast cancers by detecting metal-bearing antibodies injected into the patient's bloodstream. These antibodies concentrate at the tumor site, where they are recorded by radiomagnetic signals. However, scientists feel the equipment is not thorough enough, and is prohibitively expensive.

Magnetic Resonance Imaging is perhaps most important in detecting metastatic breast disease, and is particularly useful in detecting such conditions where the spine is involved. Whereas routine x-rays and bone scans can be negative, the MRI can be positive.

Radioisotopes

Radioactive forms of iodine, gold, and other substances are now widely used in diagnosing cancer in certain organs, such as bone, liver, and thyroid gland. These radioactive elements tend to concentrate in specific areas, making it easier for doctors and radiologists to detect and diagnose tumors. Radioisotopes are particularly helpful in determining whether a malignant tumor has spread to another organ. And since breast cancer frequently spreads to bone, radioisotopes can be used to determine if a metastasis has occurred.

Immunocytochemistry[51]

The technique of using monoclonal antibodies in diagnosis and treatment has tremendous potential, and immunocytochemical techniques have now been developed to detect cancer cells that have spread from the breast to the lymph nodes in the armpit (the most common site of metastases). Monoclonal antibodies have been used, making the technique much more accurate. If the glands prove negative for cancer, no further treatment is necessary.

SUMMARY

Many techniques have been tried in the past to image the breast effectively. But the purpose of imaging remains the same: to detect breast cancer in its earliest form. New methods are evolving: transillumination, ultrasound, and magnetic resonance imaging are a few promising ones that are still inadequate for determining benign from malignant lesions. Mammography is still the best method for finding small cancers.

Manufacturers have improved x-ray machines so that the risk of exposure of the breast to ionizing radiation has been greatly reduced. The result is that smaller and smaller cancers are located earlier and more women are qualifying for breast conservation methods.

QUESTIONS

Q. Why aren't more mammograms done? Why isn't there mass screening of the more than 40 million women in this country who are old enough to have mammograms?

A. The main reason is the cost, which would exceed several billion dollars. Mammography today is still selective and it should be. However, it should be used in all high-risk patients. Until its use is more pervasive breast self-examination remains the best option. It costs nothing, and with practice, a woman can detect lumps as small as three-quarters of an inch.

Q. Is there a best time to have a mammogram?

A. Not really. Some radiologists prefer to do mammograms in relationship to the menstrual cycle. But I find if the woman has a breast problem, the sooner it's done, the less anxiety she has.

Q. What about older patients who need mammograms?

A. They should have one yearly, if they are in a risk group. You should consult your doctor about this, however, or contact your local branch of the American Cancer Society.

Q. Are women apprehensive about mammograms?

A. Yes. Most patients who have mammograms are apprehensive and it can help if the technician is a woman and takes time to explain the procedure.

Q. Is there a limit to the number of mammograms a woman can have?

A. Yes. Screening mammography may be helpful in early detection of some breast cancers. However, screening mammography should be reserved for the risk period (after 38 years of age). The exposure of the young breast to radiation increases the risk of getting breast cancer later in life.

Q. Are all women willing to have mammograms?

A. No. Mammograms are intimidating to some women; like many of us, they're afraid of the unknown. And, too, it's sometimes an uncomfortable exam and repeated mammograms do have a slight damaging effect on the breast. A 77-year-old woman who had had 20 yearly mammograms had a curt reply when I told her she needed another annual picture. "Young man, if you keep doing these mammograms, there won't be any hair left on my titties."

Q. If I detect a lump in my breast, where should I have my mammograms taken?

A. I tell my patients to have their mammograms at a facility with the latest mammogram machines and the most experienced technicians.

Q. Who should read my mammograms?

A. A radiologist who is a specialist in reading mammographic films. It should not be just a regular radiologist.

Q. Are there enough properly trained radiologists to take on that challenge?

A. That's one of the problems. Some radiologists are better than others at reading mammograms. When mammography began, the percentage of accurate readings was poor. Today, it approaches 90 percent when done by a specialist.

Q. Should I get a second opinion concerning mammographic findings?

A. By all means—if necessary. Your cancer surgeon should also review the films—two heads are far better than one where your health is concerned. The clinical evaluation should be correlated with the radiologic findings.

Q. When you do screening mammography, how many patients have to be recalled to have further pictures taken?

A. In this country, it can be as high as a 15 percent recall rate. In Sweden, where radiologist specialists read all the mammograms, the recall rate is 3.9 percent.

Q. If a patient has a mammogram that is difficult to interpret, what should be done?

A. A magnification technique to enhance the image can be done and is quite helpful. Occasionally, ultrasound will also help determine if a lesion is solid or cystic.

Q. Is there some way that scientists can tell which patients should have frequent mammograms?

A. No. In the future, genetic profiles of breast patients will determine who the high-risk patients are.

Q. Are there any risks in having too many pictures (x-rays) taken of the breast?

A. Yes. No one should have an x-ray without a specific clinical reason. Every x-ray you have adds to your total radiation exposure and presents hazards that should, if possible, be avoided.

Q. What does x-ray exposure do to the breast?

A. Dr. Nathan B. Friedman,[52] Clinical Professor of Pathology at the University of Southern California, said that the permanent damage from radiation on normal breast tissue "ages it beyond its years and produces thin and atrophic (wasted) skin and distended or spidery blood vessels that may require other treatment." Other studies[53,54,55,56] by several investigators found evidence of breast cancer after x-ray treatment for postpartum mastitis (an inflammation of the breast caused by infection), pneumothorax therapy for tuberculosis, and in Hiroshima survivors who were young girls at the time and suffered no more than ten to 50 rads of radiation exposure.

Exposure to medical x-rays during infancy can significantly increase a woman's chances of breast cancer when she reaches her 30's, according to a recent study published in the New England Journal of Medicine by Dr. Nancy G. Hildreth of the Rochester University School of Medicine.[57] Another study done by the National Research Council[58] estimates that radiation exceeding 120 rads doubles a woman's chances of developing breast cancer, and the latency period can be as long as 15 years.

Q. If radiation is used in the treatment of cancer, why worry about the effects of a single x-ray?

A. First of all, no one questions the use of radiotherapy in diagnosis and treatment. It's the *amount* of exposure, how it's administered, and the damage to healthy tissues that may occur that's being questioned. Many oncologists feel that excessive radiation can be just as damaging as a radical mastectomy.

Q. *How is radiation harmful to the body?*

A. Any exposure to radiation is potentially harmful, since it can cause changes in normal cells as well as cancer cells. These changes occur in the genetic and protein-synthesizing components (DNA and RNA, respectively) of cells which are vital to our health. Frequent x-rays add to the total amount of radiation the body retains in the cell tissue.

Q. *What if a young woman under 20 years of age develops a breast lump? Should she have a mammogram?*

A. The surgeon caring for young women (less than 20 years of age) should be highly selective in doing mammography on them and should suggest diagnosis by ultrasound or needle aspiration. Failing these methods, a biopsy might be done. As with older women, the risk of exposure has to be weighed against the possible long-term risks, which are greater for younger women.

Q. *How can a woman tell if the x-ray equipment is up-to-date and gives the least amount of radiation exposure to the breast?*

A. Don't hesitate to ask about the equipment. Not all mammography equipment is monitored and calibrated regularly and the recommended limits on dosages can be exceeded. For years, Senator Jennings Randolph had been trying to get a federal bill passed requiring the government to set standards for certifying individuals (other than doctors and dentists) who administer x-rays. The West Virginia democrat believed it could prevent a dangerous situation. He stated, "There are many instances where people who give x-rays in hospitals and offices have no training." This can cause serious health problems. Not all states in this country require inspection of x-ray machines in hospitals and medical offices. In other words, if the equipment is faulty or the technician is untrained, overexposure can occur.

Radiation exposure is especially dangerous to young women and during pregnancy. Care must be taken so the unborn child does not receive excessive radiation.

Q. *Has the exposure to radiation during mammography been reduced?*

A. Yes. The newer machines emit much less radiation, making procedures much safer.

Q. What are the major benefits of screening mammography since you started doing mammograms in 1963?

A. More non-palpable breast cancers—both invasive and non-invasive—are being detected. More synchronous bilateral cancers are being detected, too. This means that in the cases we are seeing now, the size of the primary breast cancer has decreased, and as the size decreases, there is less chance of axillary node spread and the prognosis is better. We are also seeing more negative axillary lymph node dissections and fewer mastectomies. In all, more prevention has meant less pain and hardship for women when it comes to breast care.

6

Needle Localization

During the past five years, as radiologists have become more adept at diagnosing breast tumors, small unsuspected breast cancers are being detected. Sometimes magnification techniques are used to determine if a lesion is benign or malignant. The films are enlarged so smaller defects can be seen. If microcalcifications are present, magnification can determine the number of calcifications more accurately and help the physician decide if a biopsy is needed. Unfortunately, magnification does require a higher dose of radiation and therefore should only be used in diagnosing difficult mammographic findings.

Some tumors found by mammography are smaller than the head of a pencil and a small cluster of suspicious calcifications can't be felt. But once a small, suspicious tumor is seen on a film, how does a surgeon find and remove a tumor within a large breast? He can't blindly explore a breast surgically not knowing where to look.

In order to guide the surgeon to the suspicious area in the breast, a new technique has been developed—needle localization of breast tumors[59,60,61,62] (see Figure 6). A thin wire is placed into the suspicious area so that the surgeon knows what area to excise. The radiologist

Figure 6
NEEDLE LOCALIZATION TECHNIQUES

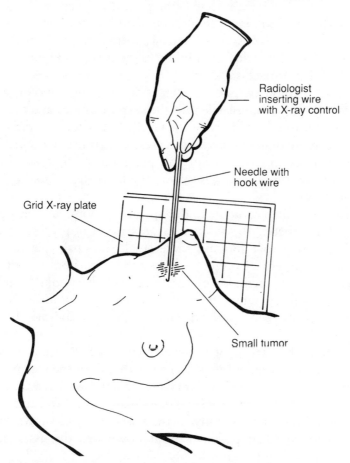

Radiologist inserting wire with X-ray control

Needle with hook wire

Grid X-ray plate

Small tumor

should explain the procedure to the patient in detail before it's done. Sometimes a short movie showing the actual procedure is shown, since most patients are apprehensive and feel convinced that they have cancer. Time should be taken to reassure the patient to assuage their fears and gain their cooperation. They should be told that most lumps are not cancerous at all, and that benign tumors can be very small and can be indistinguishable from cancer. They are also told that tumors that can't be felt are early-stage lesions, if they are cancer at all, and they would very likely be able to save the breast.

There are two needle localization methods used today. One is to guide a needle, under x-ray control, into the suspicious area and then inject a dye into the tissues to outline the area to be excised by the surgeon.

Once the dye has been injected, the patient is taken to the operating room and the surgeon makes an incision, identifies the dye-stained breast tissue, and removes the tissue for analysis. With this technique there must be no delay, for the dye diffuses rapidly in the tissue and more tissue may be removed than is necessary.

The other method, which I prefer, is to have the radiologist, under x-ray control, put a thin needle into the suspicious area and then place a hooked wire through the bore of the needle to anchor it in place.

If there is more than one suspicious area, sometimes two wires have to be used. Patients seem to tolerate this procedure well, with some reassurance, without the use of a local anesthetic. A local anesthetic can be used if necessary.

The patient is then brought to the operating room, and, using a local or general anesthetic, the suspicious area is surgically removed. The surgical approach to removing these small, non-palpable tumors depends on the surgeon. I prefer to follow the wire from its entry point and then remove a cylinder of tissue around the hook. Another approach is to estimate where the tip of the wire is within the breast and cut down over it to shorten the distance to the wire and thereby remove less tissue.

An x-ray is then taken of the specimen to confirm that the proper breast tissue has been removed. The pathologist then examines the tissue under a microscope and makes a diagnosis. Because many of these suspicious areas are very small (less than 5 mm), frozen sections of the tumor are not done. Finally, if the tissue analysis shows there is a cancer, the doctor and patient can sit down and discuss breast care options.

When a new procedure such as needle localization is introduced it takes time for radiologists and technicians to perfect their interpretation of the data. Mammography is not 100 percent accurate and there can be false-negative and false-positive readings. This means the surgical oncologist has to make the final decision as to whether a biopsy is required. If a cluster of calcifications is seen on mammography then all these lesions are biopsied. In my practice, 20 percent of patients with calcium clusters had a breast cancer, but clusters of calcifications were also linked with benign fibrocystic disease, ductal hyperplasia, fibroadenomas, and sclerosing adenosis.

PERSONAL EXPERIENCE—NEEDLE LOCALIZATION

Eight years ago, in 1983, I started to do needle localizations and biopsies on breast patients who had suspicious tumors seen on mammography. All of these tumors were tiny and undetectable by touch. At first, only a few cases were handled in this way. Out of seven cases, two cancers were detected. In 1989, 30 cases were done and ten cancers were picked up. During the past eight years, 134 cases have been done, the majority during the past four years (111 cases). Thirty-three cases of cancer have been biopsied (24 percent). The majority of needle localization cases were done because of suspicious clusters of calcifications seen on mammography. Fifteen clusters were positive for breast cancer (20 percent), and 14 cases considered suspicious by the radiologist didn't have calcifications but were diagnosed as cancer (23 percent). Three cases that had negative mammograms had biopsies and were positive for cancer.

Just what does this mean? It means that if you develop a cluster of calcifications in your breast evidenced by mammography, a needle localization biopsy should be done, as one in five will be cancer. If the radiologist feels that you have a suspicious lesion that does not contain calcium, a biopsy should still be done. If there is any doubt as to whether a biopsy should be done, the breast cancer specialist must make the final decision.

SUMMARY

Mammography continues to play a major role in the detection of breast cancer. As manufacturers of x-ray machines have made bigger and better machines that image the breast with lower radiation exposure, x-ray technicians have become more adept at positioning the patient to ensure a clear, correct image. Smaller and smaller nonpalpable lesions are being detected with magnification techniques, and radiologists reading the films are becoming more adept at recognizing the warning signs of cancer. Remember, the smaller the cancer is on discovery, the better chance there is for either a cure, or a chance for breast conservation treatment.

Needle localization of breast cancer is now being used more frequently. In this technique, the surgeon removes small pieces of breast tissue that can be examined under a microscope by the pathologist.

QUESTIONS

Q. *Does it hurt to have a needle localization of a breast tumor?*

A. Not especially. In the past four years, 111 of my patients have had needle localizations and most have tolerated the procedure without a local anesthetic.

Q. *If you find a cancer of the breast after a needle localization procedure how do your patients typically react?*

A. Initially they are upset, of course, but in most cases the breast can be saved, and this knowledge helps to ease their anxiety.

Q. *What's the biggest concern about having a needle localization of a breast tumor?*

A. The uncertainty about what will be found and whether the breast will have to be removed.

Q. *Is a surgeon present when a needle localization is done in the x-ray department?*

A. They should be present. Sometimes schedules simply don't allow for it, but I try to be there as often as possible. It's good practice, and it's helpful to the patient.

Q. *Do you occasionally get a pleasant surprise after a needle localization?*

A. Yes. Once in a while, a needle is placed into what is believed to be a suspicious tumor and it turns out to be a cyst, which is perforated and drained. The surgeon then ends up with an extremely happy, relieved patient. No surgery is necessary.

Q. *Are there some cases that make needle localizations more difficult?*

A. Yes. Women with small, dense breasts can make the procedure difficult; and women with more than one cluster of calcifications in different quadrants of one breast; or clusters of calcifications in both breasts are more difficult to evaluate.

7

Breast Lumps That Are Not Cancer

Most women will develop lumps in their breasts during their lifetime. The majority of breast irregularities are related to hormone changes that occur with the menstrual cycle. But once a woman goes through menopause, a new lump has greater significance and requires a visit to the doctor.

Until recently, more than 90 percent of all breast lumps were discovered by women themselves and the vast majority of the lumps were benign. Today more and more non-palpable lumps are being detected by mammography, but still the majority of changes in the breast are not cancer. This does not mean that you should ignore these changes. Rather, you should be aware when they occur and be expedient to investigate any newly discovered lump.

Thirty years ago, if a woman developed a persistent lump in her breast, no matter what her age, she would have a biopsy to determine if cancer was present. There were no sophisticated imaging techniques such as mammography or ultrasound to help the doctor tell if he was dealing with a serious problem. The physician had to rely on what his fingers told him in the examination of the patient. This caused extreme anxiety about the diagnosis, but in most cases no cancer was found. Today, with mammography and aspiration biopsy techniques, we can accurately predict patients who need a tissue biopsy.

In the younger age group, almost none of the breast problems are malignant. Ninety-seven percent of my patients under the age of 38 years have no serious problems. Practically all women are seen in the office, treated, and discharged. The hospital never enters the picture.

I recently reviewed the last 100 breast cancer patients I operated on. Almost 50 percent of their tumors were detected by mammography, 40 percent by the patient, and 10 percent by the doctor. The 50 percent detected by mammography were frequently minimal cancers that couldn't be felt by the patient or physician, and the majority of these patients did not need a mastectomy. Early detection of these tiny cancers meant that those patients would enjoy a much better survival rate.

FIBROCYSTIC BREAST DISEASE

Fibrocystic breast disease (the formation of benign cysts in the breast) is relatively common; 50 percent of all women experience it. Fibrocystic disease is exactly what it sounds like—an area of fibrosis and cystic change in the breast. The cysts can be multiple small cysts from which it is very difficult to obtain fluid, or large, multiple cysts which contain small or large amounts of fluid, depending on the size of the cyst.

Although the cause of fibrocystic breast disease is unknown, some studies have shown that the distinctly lumpy or thickened areas within the breast are induced by hormones. These areas typically become more prominent before the menstrual period, and are most common in 30- to 50-year-old women. Cysts are rubbery, fluid-filled sacs that can become tender, even painful, causing what many women describe as a dull ache. There can also be a sudden increase in size of a solitary cyst due to bleeding, and the pain can be quite severe.

If you have a history of cysts, you may have to have a needle aspiration to prove the lumps contain fluid and are benign. This can be done in the office under local anesthesia, sparing you the expense of a hospital stay, the risks of general anesthesia, and the anxiety of signing a consent form for a biopsy before you know what the lump is.

If you have a cyst that has been aspirated and did contain fluid, be sure to see your doctor a month later to determine whether the cyst refilled or if residual tissue is present. Occasionally a biopsy has to be done, since a tumor within a duct in the breast can cause fluid to back up and cause a cyst. What this means is that even when a cyst is found and drained, you should be religious about doing monthly breast self-examinations and keep a watch on the area where the cyst appeared. Most women with fibrocystic disease have multiple lumps in either or both breasts and will first notice change in the contour or feel of their breasts.

Several years ago, prior to the routine use of mammography, it was thought that fibrocystic disease was a precursor to breast cancer. Today, several studies[63,64] have shown this is not the case. In a review of 500 biopsied cases of proven fibrocystic disease followed for over 20 years in my practice, fewer than one percent later developed cancer of the breast. These patients' diagnoses were only for fibrocystic disease and did not encompass other pathological entities such as atypia or hyperplasia, which give an added risk.

FIBROADENOMAS

Fibroadenomas are a much more difficult problem to manage than fibrocystic disease, since in rare cases, a cancer can arise in a fibroadenoma.[65,66,67] Fibroadenomas are firm, fairly well-circumscribed, solid lumps that develop in young adult women. Fibroadenomas sometimes feel about the size of an almond or pecan and can be multiple. Most of the time they are small, single lumps but occasionally they can be very large and almost replace the breast tissue.

Since fibroadenomas are solid tumors no fluid is obtained with aspiration. If they are small fibroadenomas, it is difficult to locate and insert a needle into them. And, if found in someone older they can be bothersome, since they have to be differentiated from one form of cancer of the breast—medullary carcinoma.

The surgeon has to be careful in removing a fibroadenoma, particularly if it is large and occurs in a young woman who is still in her development stage. If too much normal breast tissue is removed, it can lead to underdevelopment of one breast and may eventually require plastic reconstruction.

INTRADUCTAL PAPILLOMAS

Papillomas are another type of growth within the breast, often occurring inside the duct near the nipple. They are too small to be felt, but are usually associated with a discharge, and are common in women in their 40's.

Intraductal papillomas usually cause pink, red, or greenish-black nipple discharge. Focused compression of the nipple area, in a clockwise fashion, will usually indicate where the papilloma is, and a discharge can be produced. Ninety-five percent of intraductal papillomas are benign and malignancy is rare. But it does occur, and the fact that malignancy does happen is a reason for excising all intraductal papillomas. If you experience this condition, remember that many papillomas are solitary, and once they are excised that's the end of the problem.

A case for illustration: The patient was a 40-year-old white woman who had been bleeding intermittently from the left nipple for two weeks. A smear from the discharge was done by the family doctor and came back Class III. The positive findings were limited to the left breast. Pressing down on her nipple area in the ten o'clock area produced a bloody discharge. Mammography studies were negative and at surgery, a small incision was made around the nipple and a dilated duct was located. A probe was passed through the dilated duct and tissue removed. The duct was then opened by the pathologist with the probe still in place and a small benign papilloma was found. This patient is now 60 years old and has had no further difficulties.

MULTIPLE INTRADUCTAL PAPILLOMAS

Multiple intraductal papillomas are a much more dangerous problem than solitary papillomas and are more often associated with cancer. However, they are not always associated with a nipple discharge. As far as I'm concerned, papillomatosis is a precancerous lesion, and patients with this diagnosis have to be followed very closely. Mammography has to be done regularly and the patient should be seen more often in follow-up since a breast cancer can develop in one of the intraductal papillomas.[68]

LIPOMAS

Lipomas are soft, benign tumors that consist of well-differentiated fat cells. They can occur singly or in groups and rarely become malignant. In fact, a lipoma may suddenly stop growing when it is no more than an inoffensive small lump with a thin membrane around it.

Lipomas are solid and sometimes aspirated with a needle but since they don't contain fluid, they may require surgery. Fortunately, they are not malignant and not a real threat to the patient. But let your doctor examine it if you find one to determine if you need a biopsy.

DUCT ECTASIA

Duct ectasia is a term used to describe an inflammation of the larger ducts within the breast tissue. As a result of the inflammation, a nipple discharge can occur and fibrosis develops within the ducts, causing blockage of glandular secretions which back up and form a lump that may be palpable under the nipple. Occasionally a watery, sticky, or bloody discharge can occur. Pain can also be associated with the lump. An advanced, often inflamed stage of duct ectasia, or comedomastitis, can also develop. The relationship between these lesions and cancer of the breast is still unclear to researchers and doctors.

THREE GOOD REASONS NOT TO WORRY

Breast Injury   Such an injury will not cause cancer, either immediately or later in life. However, a very bad bruise can cause fat necrosis (breakdown of fat tissue) which might resemble a benign tumor. If such a lump (from an injury) remains after a reasonable length of time or seems to be growing in size, see a doctor. A biopsy may be in order.

Unusual Nipples   A dimple instead of a nipple is perfectly normal, if you've had one since puberty. However, nipples that turn inward later in life can be a sign of breast cancer. If this occurs, consult your doctor. You needn't worry about an extra nipple, though. As many as 7 percent of women have one, which may be mistaken for a mole. If you wish, you can have it removed.

Asymmetrical Breasts   One breast (usually the left) is often as much as 10 percent larger than the other. If you're more asymmetrical than the usual, or if the change has recently occurred, you should see a doctor. It could be a cyst or papilloma that is causing the change.

SUMMARY

Finding a lump in the breast is catastrophic for most women. The fear of cancer casts a shadow. Those whom it does touch become so terror-stricken they are sometimes unable to fight back. Don't be one of these women. Even though the enemy (cancer) has not been wiped out, medicine is winning many battles and making great strides.

If you find a lump, don't stick your head in the sand. Seek advice from a reputable doctor.

QUESTIONS

Q. *How many patients with a breast lump who see a doctor have benign lesions?*

A. The statistics are difficult to determine because it depends on the volume of breast tumor patients seen by the doctor. In my 30 years of practice, I have seen 15 patients with benign breast tumors for each patient with breast cancer. Many cases do not come to surgery. Recently this figure has changed, however, because of the increased accuracy in diagnosis by the use of mammography.

Q. *Do many patients have an open-tissue biopsy for suspected cancer? What is the ratio with benign disease?*

A. The number of biopsies done for what is eventually found to be a benign condition continues to decrease as our diagnostic acumen advances. Interpretation of mammograms and ultrasound continues to improve as well. However, there is still a 10 percent error that persists in diagnosis.

Q. *Do all health professionals have similar skills in detecting lumps that should be biopsied?*

A. No. There is a difference in the relative ability of health professionals to detect small tumors. An experienced examiner will do a thorough and systematic breast exam and can detect small lumps that might be missed by less-experienced examiners.

Q. *Are all mammographic centers the same?*

A. No. Mammography requires a well-trained technician, modern equipment, and an expert interpreter, preferably a radiologist trained in diagnosing mammographic abnormalities.

Q. *If a woman has a benign breast tumor removed, can she still get breast cancer?*

A. Of course. The growth and development of a benign tumor is completely different and unrelated to the development of a malignant one.

8

Pregnancy and Breast Problems

When a woman is pregnant she can get a lump in her breast and the lump can be cancer. Only 1 to 3 percent of all breast cancers occur in pregnant women,[69,70,71] but because breasts enlarge during pregnancy, it's more difficult for a pregnant woman to detect lumps. This could cause a delay in diagnosis and, in turn, the development of a more advanced stage of the disease when the cancer is found. Because of the increased density of the breast tissue in pregnant women, mammograms are more difficult to interpret. Detecting a breast cancer is one of the most difficult problems pregnant women and their doctors have to face; but it is not one that should cause undue concern. Most lumps that develop during pregnancy are benign.

Pregnant women, or those who are breast-feeding, cannot perform adequate breast self-examination, nor is it easy for the obstetrician to detect any changes in the breast, particularly in the second and third trimesters of a pregnancy. If the woman is obese or has large breasts, the problem is compounded.

A delay in diagnosis should not occur simply because the patient has not checked her breasts or because the obstetrician has failed to do so. In some cases, the breasts are not checked at prenatal clinics or in the obstetrician's office. This is a bad practice. If a patient feels a new lump during pregnancy or the doctor suspects that a new lump is present, the lump should not be ignored and mammography studies should be done. A breast lump in a pregnant woman should be treated as though she weren't pregnant.

DETECTION AND TREATMENT

As pregnancy progresses it becomes more difficult to detect abnormalities in the breasts. They become firm and nodular and subtle changes can go unnoticed. There are many reasons why these changes develop. One is that the water content and blood supply of the breast increases to feed the enlarging tissue. With the resulting loss of fatty tissue, tumors are tougher to find. In the younger-mother age group, cancers are not usually present and most lumps found during pregnancy are benign. In my experience, fibrocystic disease, fibroadenomas, galactoceles, and an occasional breast infarct are the usual causes of lumps in pregnant women.

The most important consideration for patient and obstetrician is to try to detect the cancer *early.* Simply feeling the engorged breast and swollen belly is no longer adequate at prenatal checkups. The breasts should be checked during each visit. When a woman is pregnant she should persevere in doing breast self-examination, even though it may be more difficult. The obstetrician has to be both alert and aggressive in the diagnosis of breast cancer during pregnancy.

When changes in the breast are noticed and the doctor confirms them, the patient should immediately be referred to a cancer surgeon or specialist for consultation.

The initial approach when a lump is found during pregnancy is to aspirate the lesion with a needle to determine if it contains fluid (meaning it's a benign cyst) and to take a small piece of tissue for analysis. This can be done under local anesthesia with little or no discomfort to the patient. If she is apprehensive about the needle, intravenous Valium or other medications can be given so she can relax during the procedure.

Stereotaxic biopsy under radiology control can also be done.[72] If there is any question about the tissue obtained, a biopsy can be performed by the surgeon.

Even though it is difficult to establish a diagnosis by mammography in a pregnant female, it is helpful at times and should be used.

Although most imaging methods use radiation, it is possible to protect the unborn baby by putting a lead shield over the mother's abdomen, and this is done routinely in most centers. Ultrasound can also be used to differentiate between a cyst and a solid lesion.

Regardless of the method employed, the main objectives in the treatment of pregnant women with breast cancer are to cure the patient and deliver a healthy baby. This can only be done if the cancer is localized and hasn't spread to the axillary (armpit) nodes or other organs. Unfortunately, this is not always the case; in one study, three-fourths of pregnant patients with breast cancer had metastases (spread) to the axillary nodes, and required surgery.[73]

Another point to consider when taking tests is that pregnancy in itself suppresses the body's immune system and causes a decrease in the cancer-fighting lymphocytes present in the blood.[74] This change is due in part to the influence of hormones, which greatly increase during the second and third trimester. My initial approach when a lump is found during pregnancy is to aspirate the lump with a needle to see if it contains fluid (again, indicating it's a benign cyst) and to take a small piece of tissue for analysis.

The following example illustrates the difficulty in diagnosing breast cancer when the features of pregnancy mask or cause problems for the physician.

A 30-year-old woman during her first pregnancy was notified that she was pregnant when already in her third month. A physical examination indicated she was healthy and she was advised by the obstetrician concerning medications and nutrition. Six months into the pregnancy another member of the group practice she patronized examined her and detected a small lump in her right breast. She was then told to see a general surgeon who also examined her and arranged for monthly visits until she was at full term.

By then her breasts had enlarged and further efforts to see if the lump had increased in size were futile. She delivered a normal, healthy baby and asked if she could breast-feed the child. She was told to do so by both the obstetrician and surgeon who had examined her. After three months of breast-feeding, the lump in her right breast became quite obvious, and a biopsy was suggested. It revealed an infiltrating ductal breast cancer that required a modified mastectomy with axillary dissection, showing spread to five lymph nodes in the armpit. Chemotherapy and radiation therapy were also necessary.

This case history underscores several points that should be considered when a woman develops breast cancer during pregnancy. The most important is that diagnostic tests for breast cancer early in pregnancy present little or no risk to the unborn child. Second, if the cancer is detected during the second or third trimester, the prognosis is poorer than it would be during the first trimester.[75]

RISKS TO THE CHILD

If a cancer develops within the breast of a pregnant woman it's important to stage the disease accurately, and do a comprehensive evaluation of the spread of the cancer. The treatment for a pregnant woman with breast cancer is often the same as if she were not pregnant. If a woman has a surgically resectable tumor and shows no evidence of spread, a modified mastectomy and node sampling can be done. In patients with Stage II or III breast cancer, adjuvant chemotherapy is usually given. But in the pregnant woman there is the risk of chemotherapy-induced changes in the fetus.

Pregnant women with breast cancer have been successfully treated with drugs during their pregnancy and have delivered healthy babies with no evidence of toxic effects.[76,77] Others have had a simple biopsy or lumpectomy to remove a breast tumor and proceeded to give birth with no injury to mother or child. One should be careful, however, since some drugs can cause birth defects. If chemotherapy is recommended, risk to the fetus and the question of whether to terminate the pregnancy must be discussed with the woman and her husband. Chemotherapy should not be withheld because of pregnancy unless, of course, it is the woman's choice.

As to whether the pregnancy should be terminated if a woman develops breast cancer, there are no definitive answers. The question of abortion aside, it would depend on the stage of the cancer when it is found, and whether the woman had already had other healthy children. In the latter case, my advice would be to terminate the pregnancy in the first trimester and treat the cancer. If this is not possible, the mother and child should be monitored (through mammography and ultrasound) and the baby delivered early by caesarean section. This would permit aggressive chemotherapy, if needed, for the mother at an earlier date.

SHOULD YOU BREAST-FEED?

Contrary to a belief held for many years, breast-feeding is not reliable as a natural means of preventing breast cancer. Studies indicate, in fact, that a certain percentage of nursing mothers develop breast cancer and, accordingly, that the percentage rises significantly for women who are already in the higher risk groups.[78]

And there's another risk to the mother: increased hormones in the breast milk have been shown to promote the growth of breast tumors. It is known, for example, that plasma prolactin levels increase during lactation, as do the levels of estrogen and progesterone—hormones that can enhance the growth of breast cancer. Increased levels of corticosteroids and growth hormones during pregnancy reduce the ability of the immune system to fight cancer.

Prophylactic removal of the ovaries of women with breast cancer is not necessary after childbirth, as this has not proved to be an effective cure or means of increased survival.[79,80] Treatment of lactating women should be the same as that for those who aren't pregnant or who have had children in the past.

SHOULD A WOMAN GET PREGNANT AFTER BREAST CANCER?

That question has to be freely discussed with the doctor. Pregnancies are not unusual among women who have been treated for breast cancer and remained fertile. Some of my patients have delivered healthy babies following their recovery from mastectomies. If the axillary glands (nodes) were not involved, the patients seem to do very well. I usually try to encourage patients with positive glands not to get pregnant. I also suggest that node-negative patients wait at least two years after their breast cancers before attempting to get pregnant, since most recurrences happen within the first two years after surgery. I have also had a few patients with positive nodes that have not taken my advice, had a healthy baby, and survived more than 17 years after the pregnancy.

Each case has to be treated individually, and each patient completely informed concerning her prognosis. In some cases, the patient has not taken the doctor's advice and both have been pleasantly surprised.

WHAT ABOUT DES?

Before the Food and Drug Administration took action on di-ethylstilbesterol (DES), approximately four million women took the drug during pregnancy in order to prevent miscarriage. A recent study in the *New England Journal of Medicine* shows a 47 percent greater risk of breast cancer for these women.[81]

The daughters of these DES users, many of whom are now in their childbearing years, are also believed to have twice the risk of developing dysplasia and carcinoma in situ (both precancerous conditions), as well as vulvar and cervical cancer. They should consult their physician so they can be watched at more frequent intervals.

SUMMARY

Only a small number of doctors meet all the guidelines in testing for breast cancer, suggesting either unfamiliarity with the tests, or acquiescence in the face of the patient's reluctance to undergo the tests. Both reasons fail to justify the breach. No woman, especially one who is pregnant, should have to fear for her life or that of her child. An informed patient can assist her doctor by informing him or her that she is in a risk group. Any patient whose concerns are brushed aside should find another doctor.

QUESTIONS

Q. *Are most lumps that develop during pregnancy malignant?*

A. No. The majority are benign. But a pregnant woman can develop any type of breast problem that she can when she is not pregnant.

Q. *How accurate is needle aspiration of the breast?*

A. It depends. If it is done by a skilled surgeon familiar with the technique, and an adequate sample is taken, and the laboratory has reliable cytopathologists, the tissue analysis can be 90 percent accurate.

Q. *What is the most frequently asked question when a diagnosis of breast cancer is made in a young woman?*

A. The question is whether she can have children. The answer is yes. And the chances are she will do well. Seven to 10 percent of women who are fertile after mastectomy will have one or more pregnancies and the mother and child usually do well. Most studies show that pregnancy does not increase the chances of getting breast cancer,[82,83] although it probably does not protect against breast cancer recurrence.

Q. *What do you tell the breast cancer patient if she asks if she can get pregnant?*

A. If the patient shows no evidence of spread of her breast disease, I usually recommend she wait two years before getting pregnant. If she shows evidence of diffuse systemic spread of her disease, such as metastases to bone, I discourage pregnancy.

I have had a patient with greater than four axillary lymph nodes involved with breast cancer who has had a healthy pregnancy, and mother and child have done well for over 20 years.

Q. *Is it more difficult to detect a breast lump when a woman is pregnant?*

A. It depends on when the breast lump or tumor develops. If a woman develops a tumor in the first trimester of her pregnancy it is usually not difficult to determine clinically that there is something abnormal within the breast tissue. A malignant tumor is usually firmer, probably not tender, and may be attached to underlying muscle or skin. However, if a tumor develops later in the pregnancy when the breasts are larger it is much more difficult to know if a problem exists.

Q. *If a pregnant woman develops a breast cancer in the sixth month (or latter half) of her pregnancy, is it more dangerous to her than during the first trimester (first three months)?*

A. If a woman develops a breast cancer during the second half of her pregnancy she has a poorer prognosis than one who develops a cancer during the first half of her pregnancy.[75,84] Most patients who develop breast cancer during the second half of pregnancy show evidence of their cancer spreading to lymph nodes. This suggests they are in an advanced stage of disease.[85]

Q. *What if a breast lump is detected immediately after the birth of a child and the mother is breast-feeding? In other words, if the mother is lactating, and she develops a breast cancer, is the survival rate poorer?*

A. There are some who feel that lactation reduces the risk of breast cancer, despite findings to the contrary.[78] I have seen lactating women with breast lumps and if the breast is large it can be extremely difficult to detect a cancer and this can lead to delay in diagnosis. And, if there is a prolonged delay in diagnosis and treatment, the survival rate will be poor.

Q. *If a woman is pregnant and needs x-rays, should she worry about radiation exposure?*

A. Of course. She should inform the radiologist about the pregnancy, and her pelvic organs should be protected by a lead shield.

Q. *If a woman is pregnant and feels a suspicious lump in her breast, what should she do?*

A. She should have a diagnostic workup done the same as women who are not pregnant.

Q. What are the five- and ten-year survival rates for a woman who becomes pregnant following a mastectomy?

A. The same as for women who do not become pregnant.[84,85] Each case has different factors that must be weighed, including age, health, and type of surgery.

Q. What if she has a mammogram and the x-ray shows a cluster of calcifications?

A. It would depend on what trimester of pregnancy she's in as to what would be recommended.

Q. What do you mean?

A. If she's in the first trimester (first three months) I'd do a needle localization biopsy or stereotaxic biopsy of the lesion—as I would for a woman who is not pregnant. I'd tell her that approximately 20 percent of these lesions are positive for cancer but 80 percent are negative.

Q. What if she has a minimal cancer?

A. I'd probably treat her with a lumpectomy and axillary dissection if the tumor did not look aggressive. And I would withhold the radiation (5,500 R to the breast) until after the pregnancy.

Q. What if she's in the third trimester (last three months) of pregnancy and has a minimal cancer on biopsy?

A. I'd probably recommend the patient terminate the pregnancy when the baby was large enough, and then give her the best treatment I knew of. If the cancer is small, some patients might even choose to wait six to eight weeks before definitive treatment. It would be her choice.

9

What Does the Tissue Analysis Mean?

The majority of lumps, or thickenings, in the breast are benign and do not need to be biopsied. Now that sophisticated imaging devices, such as mammography, are available to the cancer specialist, fewer women need surgery. Mammography is about 90 percent accurate in detecting cancers. If there is any doubt about whether a biopsy should be done, the clinical judgment of the surgeon should prevail.

Young women who have begun menstruating have many changes in their breasts during their cycle. Some of these changes are influenced by the birth control pill.

Various inflammations of the breast (mastitis) are quite common. They may follow childbirth or injury and often become chronic, making them easily confused with cancer. They are usually not serious, although they can be very painful, especially before the menstrual period.

Breast lumps can develop during pregnancy and are usually benign. However, cancer can also develop; the pregnant woman should continue to check her breasts during pregnancy.

Cysts and other swellings occur fairly frequently in the breasts and are seldom dangerous; usually they are drained with a needle in the doctor's office and that's the end of it. Abscesses may result from infection and can be either drained or treated with antibiotics.

Most cancers of the breast are firm, solid, and increase in size. They are usually picked up by breast self-examination or are found by x-ray screening methods.

If tissue is removed in relation to any of these conditions and questions linger after it is analyzed as to whether it is cancerous, then an unbiased consultation with another medical center pathologist should be obtained.

The Armed Forces Institute of Pathology in Washington, D.C. maintains a diagnostic center to aid hospitals in obtaining a proper tissue diagnosis, and these second opinions are accessible to the patient. This is recommended however, only where there is difficulty in establishing a diagnosis. This is not recommended for the routine breast cancer case.

There are many factors that determine the fate of the breast cancer patient: the size of the primary tumor, the type of tumor present on tissue analysis, whether or not the lymph nodes are involved with spread of the cancer, the steroid hormone receptors, whether the cancer has entered the bloodstream and involved the bones or other organs, the menopausal status of the patient, and the patient's own ability to resist the cancer. There are other factors, but these are the important ones.

Staging systems—or techniques to determine the extent of the cancer—have been devised and used prior to treatment, and are often found to be inaccurate. Analysis of the tissue, by a pathologist, is still the best method to determine extent of disease.

The importance of the tissue analysis of the breast tumor and the glands under the armpit cannot be overemphasized, for it is the analysis of this tissue that will direct the proper treatment, if further treatment is necessary. *The single most important factor in relationship to prognosis is whether the axillary lymph nodes are involved with the cancer.*

When the lump is removed from the breast by the surgeon, a frozen section or immediate microscopic study of the tissue is done. If the tumor is cancerous on frozen section, that tissue will be saved for a complex analysis and special staining of the cells to establish exactly what type of malignant breast tumor is present.

Part of the tissue will be saved to determine the content of its estrogen and progesterone (hormones). This allows the doctor to tell if he is dealing with a hormone-dependent tumor. The information is valuable if the tumor spreads (metastasizes) later on. Hormonal manipulation and/ or chemotherapy can be used to improve both the survival and the quality of the patient's life.

A few years ago, hormone manipulation was always done with surgery by removing the ovaries and/or the adrenal glands, which are where most of the estrogen hormones are made. Since the majority of breast cancers are estrogen-dependent, it was reasoned that by removing the source of estrogen, the tumor's growth would be stopped and survival time would be increased. This is exactly what happened.

Researchers working with pharmaceutical companies then developed estrogen-blocking agents (Tamoxifen), which worked just as well as the ablative surgery. This is why, if you have a biopsy of a breast tumor that is diagnosed as cancer, you should ask your doctor whether the tumor tissue has been sent for analysis of its estrogen and progesterone hormone levels.

ESTROGEN AND PROGESTERONE RECEPTORS

Estrogen and progesterone receptors are proteins in the tumor tissue, and the best time to sample and analyze these receptors is when the biopsy of the breast tumor is done.

In order for proper evaluation of steroid hormone receptors, the surgeon has to correctly perform the biopsy, the pathologist must properly freeze and care for the specimen, and the laboratory must accurately assess the material.

Analyses of estrogen- and progesterone-receptor tissue are important because they allow the doctor to select therapy that may be helpful in treatment for recurrent or systemic metastases.

The effectiveness of endocrine therapy closely correlates with the measured hormone receptor levels. Hormone manipulation seems to benefit the postmenopausal patients the best. Women who exhibit recurring diseases *after* menopause and have cancer-positive axillary nodes tend to live longer by using hormone-blocking agents (such as Tamoxifen)— if they have hormone receptor positive tumors. Simply stated, by blocking the flow of hormones to the cancer, physicians can prolong the lives of post-menopausal women. Recent research has developed a technique for determining steroid hormone receptors from fixed tissue.

AXILLARY LYMPH NODES—GLANDULAR SPREAD

The removal of the lymph glands under the armpit (axillary lymph nodes) after the diagnosis of breast cancer has been established by biopsy is the single most important procedure to determine the patient's future health.

Until recently, the number of lymph nodes affected determined what further treatment should be used (chemotherapy or radiation). This is why it was extremely important that an adequate axillary dissection be done in all breast cancer cases, even if a lumpectomy was the treatment selected to save the breast.

Doing an axillary dissection stages the disease, and the examination of the lymph gland tissue tells the doctor whether the tumor has spread. It is an excellent indicator test for the stage of the disease.

Clinical staging is inaccurate. Research studies using this method are not factual. The examination of the armpit for spread of tumor to the axilla by palpation alone is insufficient.

TUMOR MARKERS

A search for a specific tumor marker for breast cancer has been going on for many years. An attempt to find such a substance that can be measured quantitatively by biochemical or immunochemical means has been unsuccessful thus far. If we could find a breast cancer tumor marker, we could screen groups of females in the high-risk group and detect the cancer at an early stage, hopefully treating it before regional or systemic metastases occur.

Tumor markers can be enzymes, hormones, specific proteins, metabolites, or tumor antigens. Unfortunately, tumor markers are not prevalent and recognizable in early breast cancer but have been helpful in the patient with breast cancer that has disseminated. *CEA antigen*, which is a tumor marker, has been used to monitor patients with colon cancer and is now being used to follow the course of breast cancer patients with diffuse metastases. The levels of some tumor markers (like CEA) can be elevated when bony metastases or liver metastases occur.

IDENTIFICATION OF CHEMOTHERAPY-SENSITIVE PATIENTS

A search for a way to identify patients who would benefit most from chemotherapy is being undertaken in many research centers.[86,87]

There is evidence that the proliferative rate of a patient's tumor is extremely important in considering chemotherapy, as well as how fast a patient's breast tumor cells divide and multiply. This may help predict the rate of recurrence and also the survival of that patient. It's a fact that cancers showing rapid cell division, such as leukemia and lymphomas, respond best to chemotherapy treatment. This suggests that breast cancers with rapid cell division will probably not respond to just local excision, and chemotherapy would also need to be added.

A method called DNA cytometry[86] is helping identify those patients who have micrometastases at the time of the initial diagnosis. This is a step in the right direction. Only time will tell its full value.

A recent article describes an attempt at correlation of invasive breast cancer with tumor angiogenesis and metastases.

Experimental evidence suggests that the growth of a tumor beyond a certain size requires growth of more blood vessels (angiogenesis). Counting the number of new microvessels under the microscope in invasive breast cancer may be a method to predict metastatic disease in the axillary lymph nodes or at distant sites in the body—these patients would then be selected for more aggressive therapy.[88]

10

Informed Consent

What is informed consent? How does the doctor explain the various methods of treatment and the potential results of those treatments since there are many options and controversies concerning the results?

Who should define the best treatment? Some of the best researchers and clinical cancer specialists cannot agree on how the breast cancer patient should be treated. Due to the magnitude of the breast cancer problem (150,000 new breast cancer cases diagnosed each year, and 50,000 related deaths), the media has capitalized on the problem and in some cases has prejudiced the patient regarding treatment methods. Largely because of this publicity, all patients go into the doctor's office expecting to have their breasts saved if they have breast cancer.

Some of these patients don't qualify for breast conservation surgery, but an increasing number do. As I said earlier, up until 20 years ago approximately half of breast cancer patients evidenced spread of their cancer when first diagnosed (regional lymph node metastases or systemic metastases) and could not have minimal surgery. In fact, many did not need surgery at all. Other modalities were used to try to save their lives and increase their chance of survival.

Informed consent defines itself: it means the patient should be fully informed and comprehensively instructed about her options in treatment to select the method she wants. (The patient's mental competency, therefore, has to be honestly evaluated by the physician.) After being fully informed, she then consents or declines the proposed medical, surgical, or radiation treatment. She may also decide to seek a second opinion from a trained cancer specialist. In other words, she is the captain of her own destiny.

In some cases it's almost impossible to clearly explain the treatment methods and the numerous options at hand, particularly if something more than a segmental resection (lumpectomy) is to be performed. This is due to the emotional stress and anxiety associated with the discovery of the breast lump. When emotions interfere with understanding, I recommend the husband or family members assist in explaining the various treatment options.

Some states have passed laws requiring informed consent for the breast patient (California, Massachusetts, Hawaii, and Wisconsin). Other states are now considering passage of similar laws. Unfortunately, these laws have increased medicolegal problems and consequently have increased the cost of care. Some states (New York, Vermont) require the physician to discuss all options of treatment, possible complications, and risks associated with the method chosen. This means the risks explained to the patient must conform to the practice and treatment methods available in that particular community. This assumes—sometimes erroneously—the local treatment methods are appropriate for the patient and that there is some conformity to the treatment methods that are practiced nationally at major cancer research centers.

But not all major cancer research centers or hospitals treat breast cancer the same way. Breast cancer is currently treated by several different methods, demanding individual treatment for each case. Every woman should discuss *all* the options available with her cancer specialist and the reasons for the specific procedures. There is no one, standardized approach. In this book I have tried to discuss the various breast care options that are available and some of the possible risks associated with these treatment options.

The treatment methods used are considered up-to-date at the time of this writing, but may be completely different in the near future. Until 30 years ago, radical mastectomy was the treatment of choice. Today, only about 4 percent of breast cancer patients have this treatment.

One of the biggest breakthroughs affecting treatment methods during the past 30 years is the ability to detect minimal cancers with the use of imaging devices (mammography, xeromammography, and ultrasound). This means that, because the cancer is very small when detected, we can offer the patient many different treatment options and can often preserve the breast.

There are many different modalities for primary curable breast cancer. Primarily, these include segmental resection (lumpectomy) with or without lymph node dissection, and/or radiation therapy; modified or total mastectomy with axillary dissection; and radical mastectomy or extended radical mastectomy with or without radiation. The trend is definitely toward saving the breast.

Many institutions have long legal forms that have to be completed prior to treatment. I have seen some of these forms and the legal verbiage only leads to more confusion for the patient. Couple this with the fact that patients often seek second or third opinions when they have a serious breast problem, and, as these second and third opinions are in conflict with each other, the process leads to further confusion for the patient.

An average level of intelligence is necessary for the patient to select treatment methods that they can be satisfied with. Not all patients have this level of intelligence. There is sometimes a sense of futility in trying to explain everything to the patient. A patient's decision-making capacity may be altered due to excessive stress, fatigue, or the effects of medication. A relative's or friend's negative or positive opinion of having a mastectomy, or other treatment, may also influence the patient unduly.

It's impossible to inform patients completely about what will happen to them following treatment. A mastectomy patient of mine recently joined a hospital group therapy session for breast patients. The group was made up of patients who had mastectomies, lumpectomies, radiation therapy, and chemotherapy. She called me after attending the first support session. She told me she had had the wrong operation and would not see me again. She had met a woman with breast cancer who had a lumpectomy and axillary dissection followed by radiation therapy. My patient insisted I had done the wrong operation on her and that she should have had the lesser procedure, as did her friend in the support group. My patient had multicentric infiltrating ductal cancer (cancer in three quadrants of her breast).

Eighteen months later she returned to my office and wanted me to follow her again. I asked her what had changed her mind. She told me that her friend, who had told her that she had the wrong operation, died.

She commented, "Now I realize that everyone's problem is not the same." To emphasize this point, I offer the following examples about the unpredictability of breast cancer.

A patient of mine who was 59 years old had a breast cancer treated by mastectomy. Ten years after her mastectomy she developed a severe toothache and visited an oral surgeon who, while doing a root canal, noted some peculiar tissue in her tooth socket. She had no other symptoms. The tissue removed from her tooth socket was sent to the laboratory and a diagnosis of metastatic breast cancer was established. Except for this single area, there was no evidence of bone, liver, or soft tissue spread. Four months later, evidence of diffuse systemic spread of her cancer developed.

Another case was a 35-year-old white female, who also had a mastectomy for breast cancer, and two years later noted blurring and a blind spot in her vision. An ophthalmologist was able to diagnose a spread of her breast cancer to the retina and choroid of her eye. A few months later, evidence of diffuse systemic spread also developed in this case.

These two cases demonstrate the impossibility of telling where metastatic breast cancer will present itself. No consent form can predict or disallow these outcomes. Does the surgeon or breast cancer specialist have to guarantee the breast cancer patient a good result from their treatment and to be fully and permanently cured?

The answer is no. Not all patients are healthy vigorous individuals. Not all patients eat a good healthy diet, exercise regularly, and see their physician routinely for health problems. Delays in diagnosis and treatment are not uncommon with breast cancer. The patient is partially to blame, since many women don't do breast self-examination on a regular basis and don't get a mammogram when recommended. They also don't routinely follow up with their physician.

Should the patient be told there may be delayed risks to their treatment? If a lumpectomy is followed by radiation therapy, the long-term results of treatment cannot be predicted, since we are only now approaching 15 years' time to witness the aftermath of such treatment. The damage to the chest wall and breast by radiation could possibly induce a cancer that may occur 15 to 25 years after treatment. Is delayed recurrence after radiation treatment most important, or is total survival of the patient and preservation of the breast?

The patient has to participate in the decision. A woman may decide to take greater risks if she is young, sexually active, and wishes to preserve her breast. Many times the patient participating in the discussion of her options chooses to save her breast even though the risks may be greater. Most of these patients, it bears mentioning, are not able to preserve their breasts when a recurrent cancer develops. And, it's more difficult to do a mastectomy on radiated tissue and expensive plastic surgery is often required. The patient's first decision may have been the wrong one.

The question can be asked whether the patient should be told about the possibility of delayed consequences of the many surgical methods. And while this is an ethical question for doctors, I feel it should be stated: not all risks, complications, or recurrences can be anticipated; not all surgery is the same and not all surgeons have the same expertise.

INFORMED CONSENT CONCERNING SURGICAL COMPLICATIONS

Whenever a patient has an operation with a general anesthetic, there is always a small risk. Since the breast is more or less a surface organ there is not as much risk as there might be with a complicated resection of organs, such as kidney, colon, or stomach. Complications still occur, however. Not all patients are in good health prior to their operation. Some patients develop breast cancer after 75 years of age. They may have severe heart disease, lung problems or kidney disease and do not qualify for surgical treatment. Their choices may be limited.

So breast surgery, no matter what type, is not without its complications. These have to be discussed openly with the patient. Since fewer radical procedures are now being done and simpler surgical procedures have taken their place, complications have dramatically decreased.

Younger patients have fewer complications than older patients. This should be expected. It also follows that wound healing is poorer in the older age group and sometimes skin grafts are needed. Fluid collection under the skin flaps can occur, although with new suction devices to withdraw this fluid, this complication is less frequent. Occasionally an infection will develop, but antibiotic therapy usually alleviates the problem.

Radical mastectomy is infrequently done today, therefore marked swelling of the arm (lymphedema) on the side of the breast removal is likewise less common. We no longer see limitation of shoulder motion, or the cosmetic defect created by radical mastectomy when chest wall muscles are removed.

Modified mastectomy (removal of breast tissue without muscles) and axillary dissection (glands in the axilla) are still done. Segmental resection with axillary dissection followed by radiation is on the increase as more minimal cancers are detected by mammography. In some cases axillary node biopsy is not needed. Lumpectomy followed by radiation is not always done.

When these breast conservation procedures are done questions frequently asked by the patient are, "Did I make the right choice and did the limited surgery and radiation destroy the cancer? What happens if I develop a recurrence? Can I still have a mastectomy?" The answer to the latter question is yes. However, it is much more difficult to do a mastectomy after radiation treatment. Sometimes plastic surgeons have to be consulted and expensive flap procedures done. Mastectomy after conservation surgery and recurrence, however, is still possible.

INFORMED CONSENT AND RADIATION THERAPY

Until recently, radiation therapy has been considered an adjunctive treatment method for breast cancer and not a primary treatment method.

This concept has changed since a greater number of breast cancers are being detected earlier. Following segmentectomy (lumpectomy) and axillary dissection, radiation therapy is now being used as a primary treatment in an attempt to sterilize the local resected area. A higher dose of radiation and a more sophisticated technique is being utilized in conjunction with computers.

It's still too early to determine the long-term results of this treatment but there are many advocates for its use since it does preserve the breast. Again, though, complications can develop. Since higher doses of radiation are being used, the patient has to be fully informed of the possible complications or delayed consequences of treatment.

Rib fractures, lymphedema of the arm, radiation pneumonitis, and sometimes neurological deficits can develop, such as motor weakness to the hand or arm. Radiation damage to the brachial plexus (nerves that go from the neck to the arm) can be quite debilitating. Fortunately, this does not often occur.

In some sections of the country segmentectomy (lumpectomy) with axillary dissection is being done without radiation therapy. These patients also have to be informed of the possible increased risk of local recurrence. Some women are afraid of radiation and will not consent to its use.

INFORMED CONSENT AND CHEMOTHERAPY

Not all patients are fortunate enough to see their doctor for the first time with localized disease of the breast. In the report *1982 National Survey of Carcinoma of the Breast*,[1] one half of the patients (52 percent) were diagnosed with the localized stage of disease, while 38 percent were diagnosed in the regional stage with axillary node involvement that had spread to adjacent tissues. Seven percent of patients were reported to be in the advanced stage of disease.

This means that almost half the patients showed evidence of regional or systemic disease when first seen. Most of these patients saw medical oncologists after a biopsy was done and the diagnosis established. The medical oncologist was probably then confronted with discussing informed consent with these patients. Their job was not an easy one because the prognosis must be guarded.

The options for palliative treatment with radiation and/or chemotherapy have to be adequately discussed in detail with the patient who has advanced breast cancer. Since patients with systemic disease are much sicker, it is often difficult for the medical oncologist to justify the toxic side effects of the chemotherapeutic agents. Some effects are well known to the female population: nausea, vomiting, loss of hair, stomatitis, fatigue. It's understandably difficult for some patients to accept this palliative care.

Sometimes, because of the toxic effects of the chemotherapy on bone marrow (where the red and white cells are made) a suppression of all blood elements occurs. Due to a lack of platelets, which are necessary for blood clotting, bleeding can develop and transfusions are sometimes necessary. The white blood cell count can decrease, making the patient more prone to infection. Antibiotics have to be given and rehospitalization is sometimes necessary. Medicine can be given for the nausea and vomiting and wigs are often worn to cover the loss of hair, which usually grows back once the chemotherapy is completed. Fatigue and lethargy sometimes lead to depression and patients often need encouragement to continue their chemotherapy.

INFORMED CONSENT AND BREAST RECONSTRUCTION

If a patient has a breast cancer and the recommended treatment is total removal of the breast, reconstruction, either immediate or delayed, is often discussed. Either the surgeon doing the mastectomy or the plastic surgeon will place a silicone implant under the pectoralis major muscle. This is not a difficult procedure. The patient may insist on having a plastic surgeon place the implant because the remaining breast sometimes has to be made smaller (a procedure called reduction mammoplasty) and cosmetic revisions may need to be done at a later date. New reconstructive methods are discussed in a separate chapter.

Immediate reconstruction is not without its risks, and if a major complication develops both doctor and patient alike must face the consequences. That patient is already emotionally drained by the mastectomy and is not prepared to weather the emotional impact of poor reconstruction results such as the slough of a skin flap, infection, or prolonged hospitalization. In some large hospitals, where immediate reconstruction is done frequently, and with greater expertise, there are fewer complications.

Delayed reconstruction is usually recommended. This allows time for the doctor to watch the patient for local recurrence and allows the patient to adjust physically and emotionally to the absence of the breast. If a recurrence is going to develop it usually occurs within the first year or two following mastectomy.

If delayed reconstruction is done, it allows sufficient time for complete examination of the excised tissue and nodal status to determine the extent of the disease. In other words, if there is a lot of disease found in the breast or nodes, immediate reconstruction should definitely not be done. Estrogen and progesterone levels can be evaluated quantitatively so that progress may be predicted and, if necessary, future treatment planned.

Not all patients qualify for breast reconstruction. Patients with advanced breast disease with extensive lymph node metastases or diffuse bone or lung metastases, for example, would not qualify.

Patients are also told that reconstruction will not make their body image the same as it was prior to mastectomy and that the reconstructed breast, whether a silicone implant or muscle transfer, may interfere with the doctor's ability to examine the patient's chest wall for recurrent cancer. But they will be told of the positive aspects of reconstruction also. Many women opt for reconstruction to feel "whole" again, and to rid themselves of a breast prosthesis.

QUESTIONS

Q. How do you try to inform the patient concerning risks and complications of treatment?

A. One method is to have the patient come into the office with her husband or partner (grown children also sometimes attend) and discuss all options prior to treatment. This allows the family to be informed and help participate in the decision. A secretary can take notes to document the discussion so that no misunderstanding occurs. These notes can be included in the patient's chart.

Q. *How do you feel about long informed-consent forms that the patient has to read and sign prior to treatment?*

A. Long legal forms, with numerous questions, have been devised, but there is no such thing as a form that will cover all aspects of breast disease. Diagnostic methods, proposed treatment, and risks and complications that may occur are too complex to be addressed in a form. However, the patient should expect to sign some sort of consent form because of the ominous medico-legal climate today.

Q. *Would you elaborate on that?*

A. The solution is not to have a long legal form for the patient to sign. Rather there should be a complete understandable verbal discussion of treatment. However, there are many alternative methods of treatment today and we do not have a complete answer as to how the breast cancer patient should be treated in all cases.

Q. *What if the patient asks if you would recommend the same treatment for your wife or daughter if they had the same problem?*

A. I'd answer as honestly as I could. I do not object to personalizing my opinions because I want the patient to be confident in me as their physician; nor do I object to second or third opinions, for the same reason.

Q. *After the patient has been informed can she refuse treatment?*

A. Any patient can refuse any treatment if they are mentally competent, but this can be a difficult problem. I have had patients refuse treatment and then come back three months later and want me to treat them. Because of the delay in treatment the results are not as good. This type of case has to be carefully documented.

The level of fear and denial in dealing with breast cancer is such that many patients will delay treatment, even at great risk to themselves, before accepting treatment.

11

Development of Breast Cancer Treatment

One hundred years ago, practically all women died if they developed breast cancer. The high mortality rate occurred because the disease was not recognized early, surgery was primitive, radiation (x-ray) had not been discovered, and there was no chemotherapy or immunotherapy to help prevent recurrence.

Surgical treatment for cancer of the breast was introduced by Dr. William S. Halsted,[89] a Johns Hopkins surgeon, in the late nineteenth century. Halsted believed if you excised the cancer when it was localized to the breast, you could cure the patient. He also felt that cancer of the breast spread to the lymph glands under the armpit (axillary nodes) and that these glands acted as a blockage for further dissemination of the disease.

If the glands became involved, Halsted's en bloc resection of the breast, muscles, and glands (radical mastectomy) would also cure the patient. As the disease more extensively pervaded the glands, the cancer would spread throughout the body. He did not believe that cancer of the breast spread via the bloodstream.

This treatment in the early 1900's would today have to be considered both barbaric and heroic, when one considers there were no antibiotics to treat infection, blood transfusions were not available, and anesthesia was primitive. No thoughts were given to cosmetic appearance or reconstruction of the breast. Surgical complications did exist and patients were lost on the operating table—but the survival rate of breast cancer patients improved.

The operation devised by Halsted became the popular treatment for years and held out hope for patients afflicted with the disease. Before, 100 percent of the patients died, now 50 percent survived five years. Other benefits were realized from this radical surgical approach to treatment of breast cancer. The tissue removed allowed pathologists to study the various types of malignant tumors and an attempt at staging the disease evolved. Staging is the process by which doctors learn the extent of the cancer, and how best to treat it. Cancers in Stage I are localized and the most curable. Stage IV cancers are the most advanced and hardest to control. By today's standards, few of Dr. William S. Halsted's patients would be operated on because of the size of their tumors. Radiation and chemotherapy would be more practical alternatives.

About the time that Halsted was popularizing radical mastectomy, Wilhelm Conrad Roentgen,[90,91] a German physicist, discovered Roentgen Rays (x-rays) in 1895. He received the Nobel Prize in medicine for his research, which allowed the physician to look into the human body and outline its structures (bones, lungs, brain, etc.). He developed the concept of using radiation for diagnosis and then for therapy in the treatment of cancer.

Many of the breast cancers that Dr. Halsted treated, when first seen, were large, primary tumors with obvious or predictable spread. Surgery alone could not cure these women and the long-term results of radical mastectomy were often disappointing. It was not long before radiation therapy was added to the treatment of breast cancer patients.

This combined treatment method (radical surgery followed by radiation therapy) did not improve survival but did reduce local recurrence on the chest wall where radiation therapy was applied.

In the early 1940's a Scotsman, Robert McWhirter,[92] began to challenge the need for radical surgery and removal of the muscles in the treatment of breast cancer. He started treating breast cancer with simple mastectomy (removing the breast but not the muscles) followed by radiation. He declared his method just as good as Halsted's radical mastectomy.

It was soon recognized that it would be impossible to compare results of McWhirter's treatment with the radical mastectomy and radiation treatment practiced by Halsted, since no tissue (glands) was taken from under the armpit for microscopic study. It would therefore be impossible to determine whether one was dealing with local breast cancer or regional node involvement. In other words, it would be comparing apples and oranges.

In the 1960's and 1970's a growing dissatisfaction developed with the results of treatment of breast cancer by radical surgery and postoperative radiation. The five-year survival rates were not improving, and therefore medical scientists undertook controlled trials to compare the different treatment methods and set the correct course for future efforts.

After some evidence had accumulated, researchers[93,94] around the world arrived at two main conclusions concerning breast cancer survival. One, when a patient has radical breast surgery, postoperative radiation therapy does not increase her chances of survival and, two, when postoperative radiation therapy *is* given, it nullifies any advantage of a radical mastectomy over a simpler procedure (a simple mastectomy).

These findings meant that either some other method would have to be devised to improve survival, or some other type of prevention to forestall the spread of the cancer would have to be developed. Or, hopefully, both.

As a breast cancer grows, if there is delay in treatment, the problem is no longer localized. As the tumor gets larger, the cancer spreads, becoming a diffuse, disseminated, systemic disease. Exactly when this dissemination occurs is still the subject of some debate, since the methods by which a patient's body fights free-floating cancer cells (immune mechanism) has not been determined.

In other words, if you have a small tumor that is detected early, it can still be localized and the treatment results are good (either by surgery or radiation). However, if the tumor is bigger than 5 cm when first seen, the incidence of spread of the tumor is more than 50 percent. When metastasis occurs, you've got a more difficult systemic problem to solve.

In 1971, the National Cancer Institute started an in-depth clinical trial to determine if less radical procedures were comparable to radical mastectomy. Three types of treatment methods were compared: 1) radical mastectomy, 2) simple mastectomy (breast removal only), and 3) total mastectomy followed by radiation therapy. The results showed no difference in patient survival.

This study led most surgeons to abandon radical mastectomy and to use a modified mastectomy in the treatment of breast cancer. Until recently, in most major medical centers a total mastectomy (removal of all breast tissue plus the removal of sufficient nodes under the armpit) to stage the disease was recognized as standard treatment for most breast cancers (see Figure 7). However, with the increased use of screening mammography, more minimal cancers are being detected and limited surgery of the breast, such as lumpectomy and axillary dissection, is being performed more often.

Something new had to be added to the armamentarium of treatment, and it wasn't long before scientists decided to add drugs (chemotherapeutic agents) to try to increase survival rates.

A medical researcher named Bonadonna and his associates[95] at the National Tumor Cancer Institute in Milan, Italy in 1976 reported on combination chemotherapy as an adjuvant treatment in operable breast cancer. They reported improved survival rates and a reduction in local recurrence rates in the premenopausal group of women with breast cancer who received triple chemotherapy (combination of three different anticancer drugs). Something really new had been added in the treatment of breast cancer.

Recently the National Cancer Institute recommended that chemotherapy be given to all breast cancer patients whether their nodes were positive or not. This recommendation has been challenged by numerous other centers and not all centers give chemotherapy to node-negative patients.

The rationale for giving chemotherapy is that one is now dealing with systemic disease, and since surgery and radiation treatment have not increased survival rates; perhaps drugs can kill the free-floating cancer cells and improve survival rates.

The main treatments for breast cancer are surgery, radiation, chemotherapy, or combinations of the three. None are pleasant, but we are constantly finding new ways to improve surgical techniques and to minimize the discomfort caused by drugs and radiation. The balance of this chapter presents an overview of these forms of treatment and side effects that concern women most.

MODIFIED MASTECTOMY AND AXILLARY DISSECTION

The operation used frequently today is the removal of the breast tissue with a sampling of the glands in the armpit (axilla) to stage, or determine the extent of the disease.

Most breast cancer surgeons have been reluctant to accept the concept of lumpectomy or lumpectomy and radiation therapy for all breast cancer

Figure 7
MODIFIED MASTECTOMY AND AXILLARY DISSECTION

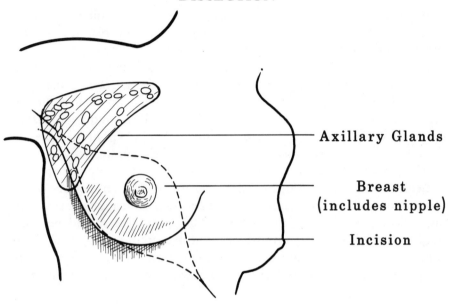

Axillary Glands

Breast
(includes nipple)

Incision

Removal of Entire Breast and
Axillary Lymphnodes – Leaving
chest muscles intact. (Transverse
Incision can be used also.)

patients because they don't want to abandon a proven method of treatment that has been in practice for many years. Stage I cancers of the breast treated by mastectomy and axillary dissection have an 80 percent survival rate and given the complexity of the disease it's difficult to imagine how those results could be improved.

Plastic surgery techniques have also improved. Immediate or delayed reconstruction of the breast with a silicone gel prosthesis has helped reduce the psychic trauma associated with the loss of the breast. Breast cancer surgeons feel that by doing a mastectomy, the risk of leaving cancer behind in another segment of the breast (multicentric breast cancer) is reduced, since a wider excision around the tumor is made. Some cancer specialists feel that to remove the entire breast for a small cancer (Stage I and Stage II) is excessive surgery and less invasive treatment, such as lumpectomy, should be used. Advocates of this method are increasing in number.

Radiation Treatment

Sometimes, after surgery, the oncologist may suggest follow-up radiation treatments either to prevent local recurrence or to treat microscopic foci of cancer in the lymph nodes.

Radiation therapy (also called x-ray therapy, radiotherapy, and irradiation) is simply the controlled emission of high-energy rays. When used on a tumor, it kills the cancer cells or interferes with their ability to reproduce, and the tumor shrinks in size. With external radiation, different units with different energy sources are used. The type of machine and dosage will depend on the size and location of the tumor, as well as the availability of the devices. Smaller hospitals may have only one unit.

Because radiation treatment is a specialized field, it's important that it is administered by a person trained and certified in therapeutic radiation (as opposed to diagnostic radiation). The technician should be thoroughly experienced in administering the maximum dosage to breast tumors while causing minimal damage to normal cells. Computers are often used to determine these factors, and treatment methods are improving as a result.

If radiation treatment is necessary, you will meet with a radiotherapist before receiving treatment. At the time of the consultation you might undergo x-rays to determine the exact size and location of the tumor (magnetic resonance imaging machines are also being used for this purpose). The tumor's position will then be marked with a tattoo (ink markings) so the radiotherapist and technician will know exactly where to direct the radiation. The number of treatments required varies depending on the tumor. Typically they will be given over a period of four to five weeks, in short sessions.

People are nervous about radiation treatment. Most fears go back to stories of horrible side effects, radiation burns, and severe nausea. Today, even with newer and safer units, women still worry. The most common question is, "Will it hurt?" The answer to this is no. But you can expect some side effects, such as a sunburned look and roughness of the skin in the area being treated. These side effects may not appear until the fourth or fifth day (or possibly later) after treatment has started. Other side effects and suggestions about self-care are included in a booklet available from the National Cancer Institute titled "Radiation Therapy and You" (see Appendix B).

If you have a small tumor that has been detected early, it can be localized and successfully treated with surgery or radiation. However, if the tumor is larger than one and one-half inches when first seen, there is a 50 percent chance it has already spread to the lymph nodes or other parts of the body. In this case, simple excision of the lump in the breast will leave cancer cells behind in at least 25 percent of patients.[96]

To eradicate the malignancy and prevent it from recurring, a high dose of radiation (5,000–6,500 rads) has to be given to the breast and suspicious nodes in the armpit. The expense is generally comparable to surgical treatment. You can ask the radiation therapist exactly how much it costs.

There are disagreements over the benefits and risks of radiation therapy for breast cancer, as with mastectomy. Several studies indicate that high-dose radiation affects the body's immune system, increasing the chance of breast cancer spreading to other parts of the body.[97,98] There are also long-term effects of prolonged exposure to radiation, such as swelling or edema in the arm.

Not everyone qualifies for radiation treatment for breast cancer. It is, however, an accepted method that is finding many adherents in this country and throughout the world. In France, for example, the treatment of choice is lumpectomy followed by radiation therapy. Every woman should discuss this option with her doctor as well as the types of surgery and chemotherapy now available.

Chemotherapy

Chemotherapy is the use of drugs for the treatment and control of disease. While any disease can be treated this way, the term chemotherapy usually refers to cancer treatment. The aim is to either completely destroy cancer cells or in some way interfere with the cells' ability to reproduce. It's believed that anticancer drugs alter the cancer cells' ability to divide and survive.

Different families of drugs are used in chemotherapy. Some are highly toxic alkylating agents (cytoxan) that short-circuit messages directing cell division. Some are antimetabolites (methotrexate, 5-fluorouracil) that kill cancer cells by mimicking substances required for cell growth. Some are extracts of plants which act as antibiotics (actinomycin, mitomycin) to disrupt the myriad functions of cancer cells. A fourth category of anticancer drugs (vinblastine, vincristine) inhibit construction of proteins vital to cell division.

Because the side effects of these drugs can be serious, the physician must maintain a delicate balance between dose and results of treatment. He strives to give sufficient chemotherapy to kill cancer cells without permanently destroying too many normal tissues. Individuals also tolerate drugs differently, so any unexplained reaction should be reported to your doctor immediately. When treatment is stopped, most side effects including anemia or hair loss disappear. To cope with the loss of appetite (common among patients receiving chemotherapy and radiation treatment), guidelines and food tips are available in the booklet "Nutrition for the Cancer Patient" that can be obtained from the U.S. Department of Health and Human Services (see Appendix B).

Rapidly growing cancer cells are most vulnerable to chemotherapy, and chemotherapeutic drugs injure cancer cells more than normal cells. But chemotherapy also suppresses the immune system, and one serious side effect is the suppression of bone marrow, which is vital to the production of white and red blood cells. Anticancer drugs and radiation can severely impair the immune system and even cause new cancers in some patients. There is substantial evidence that certain drugs affect the liver and kidneys, further limiting the body's natural response to diseases, including cancer. To prevent serious side effects, your physician can perform special blood tests to monitor how the anticancer drugs are affecting you.

Most chemotherapy is given on an outpatient basis in the doctor's office or hospital. However, for some patients, short periods of hospitalization may be necessary to monitor treatment. Before chemotherapy begins, the physician should explain reactions that might occur during the administration of specific drugs. You should ask for any available literature on the topic. Information about drugs is now available in free, easy-to-read leaflets put out by the American Medical Association, which are distributed through doctors.

Other Forms of Treatment

In addition to radiation and chemotherapy, several newer forms of treatment are being offered to breast cancer patients. Some, like lipid vesicles, are still very much in the experimental stage. Others, including hormonal manipulation, are emerging as important therapies in the management of patients with breast cancer. The principal new treatments are:

Hormone Therapies   Hormonal therapy may provide prolonged control of breast cancer for many women. This is why, whenever a breast biopsy is done and a cancer detected, the tissue should be analyzed for estrogen and progesterone binding. If the tumor tissue binds estrogen or progesterone, shrinkage or disappearance of the cancer may occur with hormonal manipulation and the cancer may go into remission for long periods of time. In fact, the National Institute of Health (and other organizations)[99] have recently endorsed hormonal therapy with the drug Tamoxifen as a preferred treatment for many older women with regional disease spread. Tamoxifen is a hormone-blocking drug that induces a sort of chemical oophorectomy (removal of ovaries). It is not recommended for women of childbearing age.

Immunotherapy   Several methods are being used, all of which show promise in the treatment of breast cancer. In one area of immunotherapy, chemically altered tumor cells are used to stimulate an anticancer response in the body. Another method is to use antibodies harvested from one person to fight cancer in another. A third method involves the injection of substances that may trigger natural anticancer mechanisms.

Hyperthermia   This is not entirely new. Deliberately inducing a high fever was used to treat cancer patients 60 years ago. Today, computer-controlled hyperthermia uses heat-producing energy to attack cancer cells selectively. In tests on patients who have failed to respond to conventional therapy, researchers have found hyperthermia treatment, when combined with radiation therapy, twice as effective as radiation alone. Immersing the patient in hot water baths also appears to increase the effectiveness of chemotherapy and radiation, according to the National Cancer Institute.

Lipid Vesicles   These are microscopic fatty capsules that deliver anticancer drugs directly to the tumor, bypassing other tissues and thereby reducing harmful side effects. When injected into the bloodstream, the vesicles release the drug at the precise place where it can be most effective. Another method uses antigens to activate the immune response of normal cells, putting them "on guard" as the vesicle passes by en route to the tumor site.

Interferon   This is possibly the most important agent in stimulating the body's immune system. Interferon has been shown to stop the spread of cancer in animal experiments, and certain tumors in humans.[100,101]

Interferons are natural substances, originally described as antiviral proteins, that are induced by viral infections in certain blood cells and fibroblasts. It's felt they potentiate, or increase, the effect of chemo-therapeutic agents.

Interferons are being used in hairy cell leukemia, endocrine pancreatic cancer, Hodgkins lymphoma, Kaposi's sarcoma and numerous other tumors on an experimental basis. The high cost and short supply of interferons has hindered research.

Photoradiation For this experimental treatment, a patient is given a photoactive material intravenously. The material accumulates in the tumor area and surrounding tissues, where it can be activated by the use of a laser beam, destroying the cancer cells. Other new methods of treating breast cancer may also be available to some patients. Ask your physician if such a program exists in your area and if you qualify.

SUMMARY

In spite of what you read in newspapers and magazines and hear on television and radio, one of the most common operations used today in the treatment of breast cancer is removal of the breast (modified mastec-tomy) and a sampling of the glands in the armpit (axillary dissection) to stage the disease.

With new imaging devices (mammography, xeromammography, ultra-sound), more minimal breast cancers are being detected before a woman can feel the lump. The percentage of breast cancer patients who now qual-ify for limited surgery has increased dramatically during the past five years (35 percent) and is still increasing. Treatment for this type of breast cancer and the related controversies are discussed in the following chapters.

12

In Situ Cancer

"You're going to need a breast biopsy." These are dreaded words for a woman to hear. Today, one in nine women will be told that a breast biopsy is cancer. The increasing accuracy of mammography in identifying lesions means fewer unnecessary open biopsies are being done by the surgeon. If the lesion is large enough to be felt, a needle biopsy that takes a small piece of tissue from the tumor can often be done in the doctor's office. Another method is to place a thin wire under x-ray control into very small, suspicious tumors and have a surgeon remove the tissue around the wire in order to establish a diagnosis.

Three to five days after the needle biopsy is done the patient meets with her breast surgeon and is sometimes told, "You have a very tiny cancer in your breast."

The apprehension of waiting for a diagnosis is over and the apprehension over therapy begins. "Can I save my breast?" is the question often asked.

"That depends on the review of the tissue and if you want to," is the reply given by the doctor.

The breast cancer specialist is not being needlessly circumspect here.

He is talking about a type of breast tumor that is seen more often because of the increased sophistication of our diagnostic acumen.

There is a condition called in situ breast cancer that an increasing number of women are diagnosed with following breast biopsy. The reason in situ breast cancer is being found is because modern mammographic techniques are detecting smaller and smaller cancers that can't be felt on palpation.

The dialogue might continue with another commonly asked question: "If the tumor is so small, does it really have to be removed?"

The answer to that question is, "If you leave it there it will continue to grow and as it grows the chance of it spreading to other vital areas in the body increases."

"How can you be sure of that?"

"Studies over the past few years show that serial mammograms can clearly show that small tumors can turn into bigger tumors that are deadly."

"I don't understand what you mean by in situ cancer. What kind of in situ breast cancer do I have?"

"There are two main types of in situ breast cancer that are diagnosed under the microscope—intraductal in situ breast cancer or lobular in situ breast cancer. They are two distinct different entities and should be treated as such."

In order to understand the terminology, a brief discussion of the anatomy of the breast will help explain what is meant by in situ intraductal or in situ lobular carcinoma of the breast.

Figure 8 shows how the breast is made up of lobules and ducts. The enlarged diagram depicts an in situ ductal carcinoma and an in situ lobular carcinoma.

A normal developed breast is made up of lobules (glandular structures) and 24 connecting milk (lactiferous) ducts that join together to form a milk sinus at the nipple. When a woman is pregnant her breast lobules produce milk that passes through the ducts to the nipple.

The two types of in situ carcinoma are two separate entities—one involves the glandular structure (lobular) and the other involves the draining (ductal) structures.

The medical term in situ cancer means that the cancerous tumor is still localized within the lobule of the breast or within the lumen of the duct and has not broken through those structures to invade surrounding tissues.

One thing to remember is that in situ cancer of the breast is considered

Figure 8
INTRADUCTAL IN SITU AND LOBULAR IN SITU CANCER

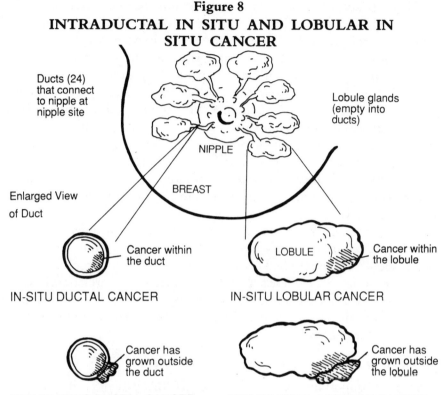

a rare condition and makes up less than five percent of all breast cancers, although with early-detection methods, more and more carcinomas in situ are being found.

In situ carcinoma is the earliest detectable type of breast cancer and, if treated properly, the prognosis can be excellent. It is considered a non-invasive cancer, or in other words, it is a small local cancer that has not affected surrounding tissue, glands, or other body structures. Most specialists feel that it's a pre-invasive cancer that eventually will spread if left unchecked.

Unfortunately, there were no studies of in situ breast cancer done long enough ago that their results might be useful to outline new treatment methods.

At the present time, the National Surgical Adjuvant Breast Project is trying to collect enough cases to compose a study that will determine optimal treatment. Yet, most scientists feel that it will take 10 to 20 years to produce statistical data that will be meaningful.

There are some pathologists who feel that intraductal carcinoma of the breast begins with the development of atypical cells that multiply and cause hyperplasia in the lining of the ducts; hyperplasia then develops into non-invasive cancer (carcinoma in situ) that eventually breaks out to form an invasive intraductal cancer capable of spreading.

This is one of the reasons that multicentricity has to be considered when talking about in situ carcinoma of the breast. The question is, if the changes are occurring in one small area of the breast (in situ cancer) why aren't the changes occurring in other areas of the breast that have not been biopsied? Might there be two or more separate foci of in situ carcinoma developing in that breast? The same stimulus creating one area of in situ cancer could be creating other areas. This is the troubling question of multicentricity.

Some pathologists feel that if in situ carcinoma of the breast is seen by looking at one microscopic slide, several sections of the surrounding tissue should also be studied because of the possibility of multicentricity. In fact, in some cases where a diagnosis of intraductal carcinoma in situ is established, further sectioning of surrounding tissue yields a diagnosis of invasive intraductal carcinoma. This drastically changes the method of treatment for that patient.

Treatment of Intraductal Carcinoma In Situ

The most important question is whether the patient, who has been diagnosed as having intraductal carcinoma in situ, will eventually develop an invasive intraductal cancer capable of spreading to lymph nodes or other vital structures that will become a threat to her life. If the in situ carcinoma does not change, then local excisional treatment is all that is needed—in other words, an excisional biopsy with adequate margins. If the in situ carcinoma progresses rapidly to form an invasive intraductal carcinoma, a more aggresssive method of treatment is necessary.

From retrospective studies, it is known that in situ ductal carcinoma can take many years to progress to invasive cancer. Some studies show that it takes 10 to 20 years before it becomes invasive. But does this mean that the patient should wait until invasive cancer develops?

An early study of 25 patients with ductal carcinoma in situ was done at Sloan Kettering by Dr. Farrow.[102] These patients were treated by excisional biopsy, and 20 percent of them later developed invasive cancer in the area of the original biopsy within eight years. This suggests either that adequate margins around the in situ cancer were not taken or that there was multicentric cancer next to the site of the original biopsy. Since this study comprised only a small number of cases, it is difficult to apply it to today's treatment methods.

In some centers, intraductal carcinoma in situ has been treated by lumpectomy followed by radiation treatment, which seemed to cut down on the local recurrence.[103] Other centers have done a total mastectomy with or without reconstruction and reported excellent results.[104]

Studies of intraductal carcinoma in situ in which axillary node dissections have been done show little evidence of metastases to the lymph nodes.[105] Therefore an axillary dissection is usually not required in this type of case, although nodal metastases have been reported in a few isolated instances.

I was recently involved with a case of intraductal carcinoma in situ in which the biopsy did not have adequate margins. A re-excision was decided upon, since the patient wished to preserve her breast. The second excision for margins showed an infiltrating ductal carcinoma within the second biopsy specimen. Because of this finding, the patient had a third operation—a modified mastectomy and axillary dissection which showed positive lymph nodes. The patient was then treated with chemotherapy.

LOBULAR CARCINOMA IN SITU

Lobular carcinoma in situ acts differently than intraductal carcinoma in situ. It is usually not picked up by mammography. Most often it is a nonpalpable lesion that is found on biopsy associated with some other process. The diagnosis, made by the pathologist, can sometimes reveal microcalcifications or sclerosing adenosis.

Lobular carcinoma in situ is considered a less lethal lesion than intraductal carcinoma in situ since many of the tumors do not develop into invasive cancer and if they do, it usually takes a long time to develop.

In my experience, lobular carcinoma in situ is most often found in premenopausal women,[106,107,108] although it has been suggested that as many as one-third of the lesions occur in the postmenopausal woman.

When a mastectomy is done, lobular carcinoma in situ is usually found in more than one quadrant of the breast. It is therefore considered multicentric and often bilateral. The figures for bilateral involvement of the breast[108,109,110,111] range from 10 percent to 35 percent and the development of invasive cancer ranges from 5 percent to 35 percent, often depending on the length of the study. In many cases it takes as long as 16 to 20 years before invasion develops.

There are several studies supporting the belief that excisional biopsy is all that is needed in the treatment of lobular carcinoma in situ. Dr. Haagensen from Columbia Medical School supported this practice and advocated frequent follow-ups (at intervals of four months) since mammography does not seem to be helpful in making the diagnosis.[107] Total mastectomy also has been done in the past with low recurrence rates.[112,113] Reconstruction is often done in some of these patients, particularly the younger premenopausal group. In some centers hormonal blocking agents (Tamoxifen) are given to help prevent recurrence.

An interesting case of lobular carcinoma in situ: The patient was a 35-year-old female who, seven years ago, noticed a small lump underneath the nipple of the right breast. A mammogram showed some calcifications in the area and a biopsy was done. The finding was lobular carcinoma in situ in a small focus. The patient was offered a mirror-image biopsy in the opposite breast but refused. No further surgery was done. Recently she was placed on Tamoxifen. She has been followed with annual mammograms and has shown no evidence of active disease.

SUMMARY

Intraductal carcinoma in situ and lobular carcinoma in situ are two separate entities. With the increased use of screening mammography, intraductal carcinoma in situ is being seen more often and is considered a marker for pre-invasive cancer. In contrast, mammography is of limited value in detecting lobular carcinoma in situ, which can remain dormant for long periods of time before becoming active. This often allows the patient to preserve her breast after excisional biopsy.

The treatment of intraductal carcinoma in situ has to be somewhat more aggressive, even though spread to the axillary lymph nodes (glands under the armpit) rarely occurs. The time interval from diagnosis to invasive cancer is much shorter than for lobular carcinoma in situ, and mammography can be helpful in detecting the progression of the disease.

QUESTIONS

Q. When you take a sample (biopsy) of the breast and the pathologist tells you that the patient has intraductal carcinoma in situ, how do you treat that patient?

A. First, I review the breast tissue slides with the pathologist. I look at the high-power field to see how many disease changes are in the ducts.

Q. *How does that help you?*

A. If there are a lot of changes in the ducts (intraductal carcinoma in situ) and it appears that free margins can not be obtained, I recommend a mastectomy. Immediate reconstruction or delayed reconstruction can be done.

Q. *Do you ever do a local excision?*

A. Yes. I recently had a patient that showed only one or two changes in the ducts in a high-power field under the microscope. I discussed it with the patient and we chose to monitor her condition with mammography at six-month intervals.

Q. *What do you tell a patient who has a lobular carcinoma in situ of the breast?*

A. I tell the patient that she has the lowest grade of cancer in her breast lobules and that she can preserve her breast with an excision of the area. The margins of excision must be clear, however. She is also told that she has to be followed at frequent intervals for the rest of her life (four-month intervals). It's vital that she share in the responsibility of preserving her breast since she may get an infiltrating cancer 10 to 20 years later.

Q. *What if you do a biopsy of the breast that is diagnosed as in situ lobular carcinoma and the margins aren't free?*

A. I usually advise a wider excision or segmentectomy to get around the lesion.

Q. *Why not just watch the patient?*

A. Because sometimes areas of in situ carcinoma occur in association with a pre-existing invasive lesion nearby.

Q. *Do you ever do an axillary dissection for in situ ductal or in situ lobular carcinoma?*

A. Not usually, because the glands are very rarely involved. However, sometimes the patient will insist on a biopsy of the glands.

Q. *Instead of using surgery (mastectomy) for the treatment of intraductal carcinoma in situ, why not use radiation therapy to preserve the breast?*

A. Some recent studies using radiation have shown a high incidence of recurrence. Therefore we may risk, in a small percentage of patients, converting a surgically curable disease into an incurable one.[114]

13

Limited Surgery

The words lumpectomy, segmentectomy, minimal surgery, and limited surgery are terms now recognized all over the world—particularly by those women who have experienced a breast biopsy and had to face cancer therapy.

During the past century, the transition from radical mastectomy to simple mastectomy with radiation, to modified mastectomy, to lumpectomy and axillary dissection followed by radiation, has marked the advancement of breast cancer therapy.

The development of x-ray equipment (mammography) has played a major role in that change as well. Mammography now detects 50 percent of breast cancers, many of them small, nonpalpable tumors. This usually qualifies the patient for new breast care options that allow for the preservation of the breast.

There no longer is just one operation—radical mastectomy—to offer the patient, and many women no longer have to fear amputation of the breast and its emotional and psychological effects.

Because many breast cancers now being detected cannot be felt, breast cancer specialists are treating a new type of patient. Prior to the development of imaging devices, almost all breast cancers were detected by breast self-examination (80 percent) and cancers that could be felt were larger and more advanced.

For women with breast cancer in the early stages (Stage I and Stage II), limited surgery followed by radiation works as well as removal of the entire breast. This gives hope to all women who are fortunate enough to be diagnosed with a small breast cancer.

Minimal cancer means there is just a small amount of cancer present that usually does not involve the lymph glands. Minimal cancer, nevertheless, sometimes can evidence early invasive features and there is still controversy as to the best method of treatment.

In some European countries lumpectomy and axillary dissection to determine spread of the cancer, followed by radiation, is the treatment of choice. In 1976, the National Cancer Institute began a comparative study to see which was the best treatment of a small cancer, since survival rates were not increasing with the standard modified mastectomy and axillary dissection. The comparison was between total removal of the breast tissue with two limited surgeries—segmentectomy (lumpectomy) with sampling of the glands in the armpit (axillary nodes), and segmentectomy with sampling of the glands and added radiation therapy after the surgery was done.

In 1985, Dr. Bernard Fisher, who led the study, and others[115] showed there was no difference in survival rates among the three groups. This meant that it was not necessary to remove the breast in Stage I and Stage II cancers. There was another interesting finding, however. The addition of radiation therapy was important because there was a marked reduction in reappearing cancer in those patients who received x-ray treatment after limited surgery. More recent evaluation of statistics by the National Cancer Institute support this finding.

The technique of limited surgery removes only the breast lump with the tumor and adjacent tissue around the cancer to obtain tissue margins, which are then studied. In addition to the partial breast surgery, a sampling of the glands under the armpit (axillary dissection) is taken to see if the cancer has spread to the lymph nodes (see Figure 9). This allows proper staging of the disease and helps determine whether the patient will need radiation therapy to treat any glandular cancer. She may also need some form of chemotherapy to try to destroy any cancer cells that may be in the body's systemic circuit.

Figure 9
SEGMENTECTOMY (LUMPECTOMY) AND AXILLARY GLAND REMOVAL

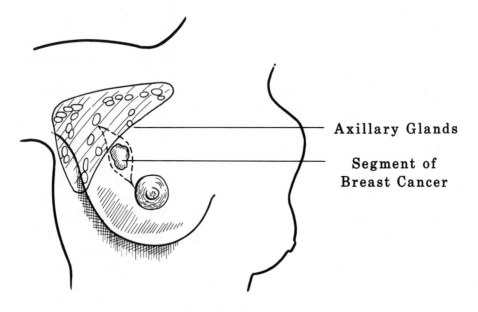

Axillary Glands

Segment of Breast Cancer

● Preserves Breast Contour.
● Radiation Therapy given after Surgery.

Radiation therapy is given to the breast after the lumpectomy is done to cut down on local recurrence and to destroy any other possible foci of cancer that may be developing (multicentric cancer).

Recent research from the National Surgical Adjuvant Breast Project[115] proposes that limited surgery (segmentectomy) does work on small breast tumors (less than 4 cm in size).

In the past, before the acceptance of mammography almost 50 percent of women, when first seen with breast cancer, presented a tumor that had already spread to the lymph glands or other parts of her body. In many cases mastectomy was the more appropriate treatment. Unfortunately, at that time—and today—not every woman with a breast cancer qualifies for breast conservation surgery. This is the hardest part for a woman to accept.

It is important to remember that each case has to be individualized prior to treatment. Not all breast cancers are the same size or progress in the same way. Many variables have to be considered, and since there are many different breast care options today, there is mass confusion as to which method is the best.

Limited surgery *does not work* if the woman is afflicted with a large, neglected cancer of the breast similar to the type that Halsted[89] took care of many years ago with his radical method of treatment.

We are now in a transition period that transverses the supraradical operations and employs modified mastectomy and breast conservation operations, such as lumpectomy and axillary node sampling, to stage the disease. The scientific community is assessing and comparing the new methods of treatment with the older methods.

We understand the malady well enough now to see there is no one approach suited to the needs of all patients. The decision regarding the extent of the surgical procedure, the use of radiation, or any other treatment must be based on extensive diagnostic studies. Other factors to consider are the type of cancer reported by the pathologist, the patient's age, and her preference in conjunction with the considered judgment of the cancer surgeon.

The choice of treatment should be one the patient fully understands. There are now a variety of telephone medical services, approved by medical societies and hospitals, that provide expert and confidential advice on medical problems, including cancer. The best of these for breast cancer is Cancer Information Service (800-638-6694), which was started by the National Cancer Institute.

To help women make an informed choice about breast cancer treatment, the rest of this chapter summarizes the different types of limited surgery and tells how they differ from modified or radical mastectomy. A discussion of the controversies is presented in a question–and–answer dialogue at the end. All women are encouraged to discuss with their physicians the available options, the details of the recommended approach, and the reasons for a specific procedure.

LUMPECTOMY

The term "lumpectomy" is not an accurate one. It is essentially only a biopsy of the tissue to see if a cancer is present. The term can be interpreted in many ways, depending on the philosophy of the operating surgeon. It can be a simple excision of the tumor, or a wide, extensive excision that may deform the breast. The placement of the incision is very important if further surgery is contemplated or plastic reconstruction is anticipated.

Women who are very thin or who have small breasts are often unhappy with the cosmetic results of a lumpectomy and it probably should not be done in those patients. It is also not universally successful if the tumor is under the nipple or deep within the breast tissue. It also bears mentioning that when a lumpectomy is done, a separate incision usually has to be made to sample the glands in the armpit for staging purposes.

SEGMENTECTOMY

A segmentectomy is usually a wider excision than a lumpectomy. It often includes the fascia (muscle covering) of the chest muscle. Four or five samples of tissue around the breast cancer are taken to be sure adequate margins are obtained. The margins are stained with different colored dyes so the pathologist can identify any possible adjacent area of involvement. Since the majority of breast cancers are in the outer quadrant of the breast, a single incision can often be made so that a sampling of the glands can be done at the same time and very limited cosmetic changes are seen in the breast (see Figure 9).

The advantages of a lumpectomy or segmental resection are that the breast is normally left intact. In fact, in some parts of the country, no further treatment is given except that the glands under the armpit may be sampled to see if they are free of tumor spread. Because of the high local recurrence rate,[116,117] most centers give postoperative radiation if a lumpectomy or segmentectomy is done. There are still some cancer centers that do not give radiation after lumpectomy if the tumor is smaller than 2 cm.

AXILLARY DISSECTION (Sampling of the axilla glands)

Sampling the glands is recommended if the tumor is greater than ½ cm in size so that both patient and doctor know the extent of the disease (unless the diagnosis is in situ carcinoma). If the tumor has metastasized to the glands, the treatment is more aggressive. The recent decision to recommend chemotherapy to all patients (node-negative) is still controversial since not all patients have a high risk for recurrence. My feeling is that a sufficient axillary dissection should be done because so much depends on whether the glands are involved or not. Upper levels of lymph glands can be affected[118] and if only a cursory sampling is done, cancer can be missed. There are some cancer specialists who disagree with this because they feel that only a small percentage of patients (7 percent) have nodal involvement if the lesions are less than 1 cm in size. They feel that axillary dissections are disabling and even if recurrence develops, further treatment can be given with no change in survival rates.

SUMMARY

There is currently a debate—one that may be nearing resolution—over the type of breast tumor surgery that should be performed. There is no doubt that more often limited surgery followed by radiation is being done.

In recent trials,[115] lumpectomy and segmentectomy have been shown to be effective in the early stages of breast cancer if the treatment is followed by radiation therapy (5,000 rads). However, not enough time has elapsed to determine long-term effectiveness. Initial reports, however, are encouraging.

QUESTIONS

Q. I should think all women with breast cancer would want to preserve their breast and have a lumpectomy or segmentectomy done rather than having the breast removed (mastectomy).

A. All women do. Unfortunately, not all patients qualify for breast conservation surgery. In the past, almost 50 percent had large tumors, evidence of regional spread (lymph glands), or systemic spread (lung, bone, liver, etc.) when first seen. Today, that percentage is decreasing rapidly due to the increasing use of mammography.

Q. What does this mean?

A. It means that in the past almost one half of the patients had a delay in diagnosis and the tumors were large or multicentric (more than one area of the breast involved), and the tumor involved the lymph glands or other organs, and usually a more extensive procedure had to be done (mastectomy and axillary dissection). Radiation therapy and chemotherapy had to be used to prevent recurrence and increase the lifespan of those women. In some cases, the patient suffered from systemic spread and only a biopsy was done to confirm the tissue diagnosis before palliative treatment started.

Q. *Should a woman seek a second opinion before surgery for breast cancer?*

A. Yes, especially if she does not have confidence in the doctor recommending her treatment. There is still disagreement over which surgical procedure is best for each type of tumor. Each case has to be individualized. However, delaying any surgery for a long period of time is not recommended.

Q. *Whom should you see?*

A. You should pick your own cancer specialist for the second opinion. In some cases, you may have to go outside your local community to get the best advice.

Q. *Since there are so many different choices of treatment for the breast cancer patient, how does the patient decide what should be done?*

A. The patient should become better informed and ask questions. She must have confidence in the doctor taking care of her and should be able to communicate candidly with him or her. She should ask what size the tumor is and whether it is localized. In some cases she will not have much choice in treatment but her body is her own and she can still refuse. If she has a minimal cancer that is detected by the new imaging devices, she will have a better prognosis and may qualify for different methods of conservation surgery.

Q. *How many women with breast cancer have limited surgery?*

A. More than 30 percent in this country, although the number is rapidly increasing. In France limited surgery followed by radiation therapy is particularly common. The European countries seem to be ahead of us in the use of limited surgery.

Q. *Why are surgeons still doing modified mastectomies for small cancers?*

A. Because many surgeons are unwilling to give up a proven operation that produces an 80 percent, five-year survival rate in Stage I cancers.

Q. *Are there other reasons?*

A. Yes, they argue that breast cancer is not a systemic disease from its onset and if treated properly in the beginning, the woman can be completely cured by adequate surgery. They feel that a breast with cancer will have other separate foci of cancer developing within it (multicentric disease). This is why they argue that the entire breast should be removed. Since it takes two to eight years for a cancer to grow to a size that you can feel and detect, it will take 15 to 20 years to determine if simpler treatment methods will produce similar long-term survival rates. In short, the jury is still out on simpler treatments.

Q. *Is there any research to substantiate this?*

A. Yes. A study done by Gallagher and Martin[119] confirmed that human breast cancer is not a local process but a disease that affects the breast diffusely in many different areas. Multiple invasive nodules were present in more than 45 percent of the cases.

Q. *Does the size of the tumor determine the multiple areas of involvement of the breast?*

A. Yes. Many cancer centers[120,121] have found that the likelihood of finding cancer in more than one area of the breast is related to the primary tumor size. What this means is that a breast with minimal cancer (smaller than 5 mm), in all likelihood does not have other cancers growing in it. Whereas a breast cancer that you can feel is more likely to have other sites of cancer developing. Studies have been done that show that breast cancers larger than 2 inches have a 50 percent chance of spreading to other areas of the body.

Q. *What do the breast conservation experts and radiation therapists say about this?*

A. They argue that radiation therapy can control the primary site after the tumor has been removed and can destroy the multicentric areas of cancer which may be left behind or within the regional lymphatics. Some argue that the microscopic foci of cancer left behind can be eradicated by the host's immune system and the small cancer will not progress.

Q. *Why was radiation therapy added to lumpectomy?*

A. Previous studies[122] in which lumpectomy alone was done showed a high incidence of local recurrence. It was felt that radiation would prevent local recurrence and increase survival. Radiation is also given if the glands are positive. Chemotherapy also is often added.

Q. *Why do radiation therapists think that radiation will work following lumpectomy, when radiation therapy did not increase survival following radical mastectomy?*

A. They feel that a higher dose of radiation is now being given (5,000 rads) with boosting doses of 1,500 rads to the local site. They also feel that the newer computerized machines do a more precise and thorough job.

Q. *Are there some cancers that can be removed by lumpectomy without any further treatment?*

A. Yes—lobular carcinoma in situ. Since it may take 20 years before invasive carcinoma develops from this form, lumpectomy is adequate— if the involvement is minimal. New imaging devices should be used to pick up any changes in the status of this carcinoma.

Q. *Does age play a role in the choice of treatment for the woman with a small breast cancer (less than 1¹/₂ inches)?*

A. I feel it does. If the woman chooses a lumpectomy followed by radiation therapy and is 55 to 65 years old, I don't worry as much about delayed adverse radiation reactions that may develop. It takes 15 to 25 years or longer for a radiation-induced cancer to show up. If the woman is young (35 years old) I do worry about it, as she has more of her life ahead of her.

Q. *Are there any other adverse reactions to radiation?*

A. Yes. Patients experience skin changes from radiation and fibrotic changes in the remaining breast tissue. Tissues don't heal as well after radiation therapy, and it's more difficult to monitor these patients, because their immune systems are suppressed by the radiation. Some cancer specialists feel that when this occurs, women are more likely to get metastatic disease.

Q. *Does radiation therapy after lumpectomy change the method of follow-up for the patient?*

A. Yes, because radiation therapy produces a hardness and fibrotic feel to the breast. It can also cause calcific changes suggestive of recurrence. It means too that more frequent mammograms and sometimes more needle biopsies have to be done. Ultrasound is also being used in these cases as an aid to detect recurrence.

Q. *Should surgeons be doing more segmentectomies (limited surgery) for breast cancer?*

A. Yes, for the minimal cancers. Until recently only a select group of women with small tumors qualified for breast conservation surgery followed by radiation treatment. However, since results similar to those for mastectomy are now being found, more women are opting to preserve their breast. New x-ray treatment techniques are providing better local and regional control. I feel that limited surgery can be done successfully for small breast cancers. There is a worry about the larger breast cancers (2 cm or larger) being treated successfully by limited surgery and radiation, since the size of the tumor determines the amount of other breast area involvement and incidence of regional or systemic spread (see Figure 5).

Q. Are there any other important factors that enter into the choice of breast conservation surgery (limited surgery) versus modified mastectomy?

A. Yes. I think the size of the tumor in relation to the size of the breast is important. If a woman has a small breast and a generous lumpectomy is done to get around the tumor, then there is very little breast to conserve. In contrast, if a woman has a large breast, there's usually less problem, as she has more remaining tissue to save.

Q. Are there other situations that make breast conservation surgery less viable?

A. Yes.

1. If the patient has diffuse multicentric cancer of the breast or the presence of two or more separate cancers.
2. If a patient has a central lesion under the nipple requiring removal of the nipple. Mastectomy is then preferable.
3. If the patient has diffuse clusters of microcalcifications on mammogram.

Q. Why do some women choose mastectomy when they obviously qualify for lumpectomy?

A. Some women prefer mastectomy because it avoids a large dose of radiation to the chest wall and five or more weeks of treatment.

Q. There seems to be a controversy developing over whether or not the nodes in the axilla should be sampled if the tumor is less than 1 cm.

A. Yes, that's true. Because axillary dissections can be disabling if not done properly and there is a small yield of metastatic nodes (7 to 10 percent).

Q. How can that issue be resolved?

A. Flow cytometry is more accurate in predicting nodal involvement and will be used more frequently in the future.

Q. Can you tell if nodes are involved by looking at the breast tumor under the microscope?

A. Sometimes. If there is evidence of lymphatic or vascular invasion in the breast cancer biopsy, you can predict an increasing incidence of nodal involvement.

14

Immediate Postoperative Care

As I've mentioned before, in the 1940's and 1950's if a woman had a breast cancer, she routinely had a radical mastectomy, which would remove all the breast tissue, the pectoral muscles of the chest wall beneath the breast, and the lymph node drainage area in the axilla (armpit). In some cases, because the tumor was sizable, large amounts of skin had to be excised and skin grafts were placed over the defect. A supraradical procedure that removed the glands along the sternum (breast bone), creating a severe chest-wall defect, was sometimes done if the tumor was present in the medial quadrant of the breast (Urban procedure).

Because of the extensive nature of the operation, a vigorous postoperative exercise program was initiated immediately following the surgery to restore function and prevent disability. The Reach to Recovery Program was instituted by the American Cancer Society to prevent fixation of the shoulder on the side of the operation and forestall swelling of the arm (lymphedema). The program was not always successful. Some patients withdrew socially, so damaging was the defect to their self-image. Women who were athletically inclined sometimes withdrew from sports such as tennis or golf. Many became severely depressed.

Today, there are many new procedures used in the care of breast cancer patients—the surgical treatment of breast cancer in the 1990's has taken giant steps and the sophistication of treatment methods has been a great boon to women. Surgeons are often able to save the breast. Reconstruction, whether immediate or delayed, can help preserve a woman's dignity and self-confidence. Plastic surgery has also improved and new innovative methods are being advanced.

Mammography now reveals small cancers that cannot be detected by human touch, which means that minimal surgery is often the treatment advocated. The smaller the breast cancer, the less chance of the tumor spreading. Simply removing the lump and sampling the glands under the armpit is commonplace. And, the survival results are similar to those of the practice of performing modified mastectomy and axillary dissection.[123] A National Institutes of Health Panel of 30 specialists that met in Bethesda, MD in 1990 came to the conclusion that lumpectomy combined with radiotherapy offers patients with Stage I and Stage II breast cancer the same chance of survival as total mastectomy. In the past, 70 percent of breast cancers were detected by the patient or physician. Today, in my practice, over 50 percent are detected by mammography and usually cannot be felt by the patient.

But certain breast-cancer dictums have not changed—clusters of calcifications seen on mammography should be biopsied, and changes in yearly mammograms have to be investigated to rule out cancer.

Another unfortunate mandate is that delays in diagnosis often allow time for cancers to grow and spread. Some larger lesions require a modified mastectomy and axillary dissection. Nancy Reagan, you might recall, had a minimal breast cancer but chose to have this procedure.

The availability of these myriad options emphasizes the fact that the patient should be allowed to participate fully in her own breast cancer treatment options.

In all my breast cancer cases, a two-stage procedure is done. This means a biopsy is performed, (usually an open biopsy) to remove the entire tumor and to obtain margins on the tissue removed. The tissue is then sent to the laboratory for microscopic analysis and to determine whether the tumor binds estrogen and/or progesterone. This information is important for future reference if the patient develops recurrent symptoms; it means that hormonal manipulation can be used to alter the progression of the tumor.

Once the tissue is analyzed, a conference with the patient and her husband, friends, or family members takes place. All her options for treatment are outlined and the relative merits of each procedure are discussed. My secretary takes notes to be included in the office records. The patient is completely informed of her options and is given answers to all questions.

I've mentioned before that younger patients, understandably, frequently select a procedure that preserves their breast, while older patients often select a modified mastectomy and axillary dissection. Many older patients do not want to undergo five weeks of radiation therapy after a lumpectomy or segmentectomy. Younger patients readily accept this because, as they are probably sexually active, they know they are saving their breast.

MODIFIED MASTECTOMY—AFTER-CARE

When a surgeon does a modified mastectomy and axillary dissection, the entire breast tissue is removed and nodes are sampled under the armpit to determine if any spread has occurred.

Following the operation I usually put a wrap-around pressure dressing over the site. Tubes (Hemovacs) are placed in the wound to suction away fluid and debris; they also help to draw the skin flaps against the chest wall so that healing can occur. Pain medication is given as needed and if there is an unusual amount of postsurgical anxiety, tranquilizers are prescribed.

Once the effect of the anesthesia has worn off, the patient's oral intake improves. Good food and nutrition should be emphasized—adequate protein is needed for healing. Special diets are not standard unless the patient is a diabetic.

Early ambulation is important, and encouraging the patient to take walks in the hospital corridors is a good policy. Otherwise, there's a greater chance of vascular complications (phlebitis).

I have a conservative approach to the use of the arm on the side of the mastectomy—I do not believe the patient should exercise that arm for at least seven days. It's been my experience that early exercise of the upper arm causes the skin flaps to slide on the chest wall and adds to fluid accumulation. I want the wound to get a good start on healing before shoulder and arm exercises are done, and I have yet to see any arm or shoulder problems come up with this conservative method of care. The other practice I'm adamant about is the use of slings—I do not allow any, since the patient becomes dependent on them and her arm stiffens.

Depression following the operation is normal. But if a patient appears to be more depressed than normal, a psychotherapist may be called in consultation, and medication is sometimes prescribed. In some cases group therapy is helpful—but this should not be used routinely for everyone.

The first dressing change of a mastectomy patient is extremely important. Sometimes, if a patient is overly apprehensive, medication is given before removing the tubes and dressing. I usually tell the patient not to look at the wound, and pull the Hemovac tubes out as gently as possible. If the patient has had a lumpectomy and wants to look at the operative site, I encourage them to do so. They can then be reassured that their breast is still there. Women who need radiation therapy after a lumpectomy are advised that there may be a tanning effect on the skin from the radiation and that the breast may feel firmer.

Lumpectomy, Axillary Dissection—AFTER-CARE

Usually when a lumpectomy of a breast tumor is done, the surgeon removes enough tissue to get around the tumor. The tissue is then given to the pathologist, who stains the different margins with different colored dyes to evince the presence of cancer. If the margin is not free of cancer, the surgeon removes further tissue.

If the patient and her doctor then decide to preserve her breast, she will probably be advised to have an axillary dissection done to remove the lymph nodes under her armpit. This procedure usually requires another incision in the axilla (armpit) and should be positioned so as not to cause an overt cosmetic defect. Ten or fifteen lymph nodes are removed to help stage the disease. If all the glands are negative, the prognosis is good, since the disease is still localized in the breast. The decision as to whether further treatment should be given, such as chemotherapy, can then be discussed.

AXILLARY DISSECTION—AFTER-CARE

Following the removal of the lymph nodes (axillary dissection), a drain or Hemovac is used to remove excess fluid and debris from the site. I use a wrap-around dressing to apply pressure since the drainage is minimal with this procedure, and the drains can usually be removed on the second postoperative day. If the wound looks ok, the patient can be discharged. The wound is then allowed to heal by itself, which usually takes ten days to two weeks. Since most patients who have had a lumpectomy and axillary dissection will receive radiation therapy, a consultation is arranged with a trained radiation therapist. The patient is told that it will take approximately five weeks of daily x-ray treatments to try to sterilize the breast area of any free-floating cancer cells. Occasionally the x-ray therapy has to be stopped for a week or so if the patient gets a "radiation burn" on the skin surface. Most patients are able to tolerate the radiation treatments quite well.

QUESTIONS

Q. *Are there any contraindications to doing a modified mastectomy?*

A. Of course. The patient has to be in good enough health to have an anesthetic. Her heart, lungs, kidneys and other organs have to be in good shape.

Q. *Are there any other contraindications?*

A. Yes. If the patient shows obvious spread of the cancer from the breast to other organs, such as the bones, lungs, or brain, surgery is usually not indicated.

Q. *Do you have to give a blood transfusion during a modified mastectomy?*

A. No. With the use of modern surgical techniques and the cautery, blood loss is usually minimal. Some religious groups will not allow the administration of blood and sometimes blood substitutes are used in these cases.

Q. *If a lumpectomy is done to remove a breast cancer and the margins are not free on tissue analysis, can the patient still preserve her breast?*

A. Yes, unless she has a very small breast. A wider lumpectomy or segmentectomy can be done to get wider margins if she has adequate breast tissue.

Q. *When a patient receives radiation therapy after a lumpectomy does she get really sick?*

A. Not always. Some patients breeze right through radiation treatment. Sometimes the treatment has to be stopped for a week or two if the skin is strongly affected by the radiation.

Q. *Is the placement of the mastectomy incision important?*

A. Yes. However, sometimes the surgeon can't place it where he wants to because of the location of the biopsy scar. A transverse incision sometimes gives a better cosmetic effect, but it can't always be used. It is up to the surgeon to make the incision in the most advantageous spot, and still gain access to the area in question.

Q. Can you get an infection following a mastectomy or lumpectomy?

A. Yes, just as with any wound. Antibiotics can usually alleviate most infections. Sometimes wound cultures have to be taken if the infection persists.

Q. What is the usual length of the hospital stay for a patient who has a modified mastectomy and axillary dissection?

A. It depends. The general health and age of the patient are extremely important. If the patient has a cardiac condition or other serious illness, the stay is longer. If the patient is young and in good health the stay is usually 3 to 4 days.

Q. Do insurance companies pay for the hospitalization?

A. Most HMOs and other insurers make full payment. However, some plans try to enforce an early discharge—two days, for instance.

Q. What do you think about that?

A. I think this is cruel and unjust. When a patient has a mastectomy there is an emotional stress added to the physical disability created by the surgery. She may have Hemovac tubes draining debris from the wound. To prevent permanent psychological scars and medical complications I think mastectomy patients need 3 to 4 days in the hospital, especially considering that not all communities have efficient home health care.

Q. Is there anything new concerning early hospital discharge following mastectomy?

A. Yes, but I must say I don't totally agree with it. At the Cleveland Clinic, a study[124] from 1984–1986 concerning early hospital discharge was done—patients went home with drains in place as early as the first postoperative day. The article states that 40 percent of the patients had partial mastectomies, so that the possibility of a disaster was minimal. Home-care observation and nursing support is necessary to implement this technique, and I believe you borrow trouble when you usher a woman out of a hospital before she is physically and psychologically prepared to leave.

15

Should All Breast Cancer Patients Have Chemotherapy?

There is controversy as to whether adjuvant chemotherapy should be given to all patients with breast cancer. Some scientists feel that breast cancer is a systemic disease from its onset and therefore should be treated with drugs to kill the cancer cells that may be left floating around the body. Others feel that breast cancer develops de novo—a cell goes haywire, multiplies rapidly and gets out of control. There are arguments for both sides. The National Cancer Institute recently suggested that adjuvant chemotherapy be given to all patients, whether the lymph glands under the armpit were involved or not.

In the February 23, 1989 issue of the *New England Journal of Medicine*, the results of four studies on the administration of systemic adjuvant chemotherapy to node-negative breast cancer patients were presented. The Ludwig Breast Cancer Group reported on 1,275 patients, half of whom received chemotherapy (one cycle of Cyclophosphamide, Methotrexate, Fluorouracil, and Leucovorin). The other half did not receive chemotherapy. After four years, the group that received chemotherapy enjoyed a 4 percent difference in disease-free survival. The Ludwig

116

Group concluded that this provided evidence of the effectiveness of the chemotherapy treatment.[125]

Other major cancer institutes have challenged these findings. Dr. Charles Balch, Chairman of Surgery at M.D. Anderson Cancer Center in Houston, told a meeting of the American College of Surgeons in Atlanta (October 1989), "The benefits, though modest, are probably real for some patients. For others, high costs and side effects probably outweigh the benefits." Dr. Balch cited two other studies indicating that patients at two hospitals who did not have chemotherapy had higher four-year, disease-free survival rates (up to 91 percent) than those in the studies who *did* undergo chemotherapy.

Many other prominent cancer specialists feel that the percentage of increase in disease-free survival (4 percent) is insufficient to warrant submitting all patients to the toxic side effects of chemotherapy (nausea, vomiting, loss of hair). One prominent doctor commented, "You're not giving these women aspirin—with each dose, a woman can expect nausea and hair loss."[126] Other scientists feel that the study is too short and may be misleading because patients who took part in the National Cancer Institute study appeared to be more severely ill than the average breast cancer patient.

Other cancer specialists feel that the benefit of treatment was seen only in disease-free survival and not in overall survival.[127] This could mean that chemotherapy treatment only delays failure.

Today, with the meteoric rise of health care costs, the cost effectiveness of a new treatment has to be weighed against its benefits.[128] To achieve an increase of only 4 percent in disease-free survival, 100 percent of patients with node-negative breast cancer would have to undergo additional chemotherapy. Chemotherapeutic drugs are not cheap and the side effects are not always minimal. The 150,000-plus women in this country who contract breast cancer every year could be given unnecessary treatment, fostering an unknown, long-term result. Some scientists feel that it will take 25 years to determine the total effect of the toxic drugs on the immune system.

Before recent changes in guidelines by the National Cancer Institute, most women did not receive chemotherapy after mastectomy or after limited surgery such as lumpectomy. If a patient had a modified mastectomy and axillary dissection (to check the nodes under the armpit) and more than three lymph nodes were involved with spread (metastases) to the glands, chemotherapy was then recommended. Usually the chemotherapy was intensive treatment for a period of one year. It is now given for six months.

Nearly 150,000 women are diagnosed with breast cancer in the United States and 50,000 die of the disease each year. When caught at an early stage, the five-year survival rate for breast cancer is about 90 percent. Many researchers feel that the National Cancer Institute guidelines for chemotherapy are too broad and should apply only to the approximately 60,000 women who are thought to have the highest risk for recurrence of the disease.

Unfortunately, it is not always possible to tell which patients have the highest risk of getting breast cancer again. There are so many variables to be considered. Did the surgeon do the operation properly? Were the margins of resection free of disease? Were adequate nodes taken from the armpit to determine potential involvement? Was proper radiation given to the lumpectomy patients? Was the proper chemotherapy given when indicated?

The current criteria in evaluating prognostic factors are:

Histopathology. Was the tumor of a high nuclear grade and did it appear aggressive under the microscope?

Size. What was the tumor size? Was there skin involvement? Were the margins free of cancer?

Steroid hormonal receptors. Did the patient's breast cancer bind estrogen and progesterone? Usually if they do, the prognosis is good. If they don't, the prognosis is poor.

But some people feel that the estrogen-receptor status is not a good determinant of high or low risk among patients with node-negative disease, and that other factors should be considered. Tumor proliferative rates and DNA content also are helpful in deciding a patient's disposition. There is now a *Thymidine Labeling Index* that is helpful. One of the most important predictors is whether the nodes under the armpit are involved with spread of the cancer. If the nodes are positive the survival rate is usually cut in half.

SHOULD ALL PATIENTS HAVE RADIATION THERAPY AFTER LUMPECTOMY AND AXILLARY DISSECTION?

There is yet another controversy over whether all patients having a segmentectomy (lumpectomy) and axillary dissection should have radiation treatment after surgery.

In 1985, the *New England Journal of Medicine*[115] reported a significant difference between those patients who received radiation therapy after segmentectomy and those who did not. Radiation therapy did cut down on local recurrences, although there were no significant differences between the two groups with respect to long-term freedom from disease or overall survival.

This article has been challenged by Dr. Robert Herman of the Cleveland Clinic Foundation. The Cleveland Clinic has had an interest in breast conserving operations for over 30 years due to the early work of Dr. George Crile, Jr., who was one of the first surgeons to do partial or segmental mastectomy without radiation therapy as the definitive treatment for small (less than 2 cm) breast cancers.

At the Cleveland Clinic, margins of 1 to 2 cm around the tumor tissue are usually done. If there is evidence of multifocal disease by tissue examination or mammography, a total mastectomy is done or radiation therapy is added.

The Cleveland Clinic opinion is that radiation therapy is not always necessary when a partial or segmental mastectomy is performed on a small cancer that is adequately excised. They feel that significant numbers of patients with small, early cancers can be treated by partial or segmental mastectomy and axillary dissection alone. Their ten- and fifteen-year survival rates are equal or equivalent to those of patients who had partial mastectomies with immediate radiation therapy or to those who had total mastectomies with axillary dissection. To radiate all patients after partial or segmental mastectomy, they feel, is unnecessary.[127]

16

Management of Cancer in the Second Breast

If a woman develops a cancer in one breast what are her chances of developing a cancer in her second breast? Is the second cancer a new cancer or is it due to metastasis of the first cancer? Was the second-breast cancer found at the same time as the first (synchronous) or did it develop a few years later (metachronous)?

In today's society, the results of treatment of one breast cancer is excellent, with 74 percent of affected women experiencing a five-year survival rate. What are the five-year survival rates if the patient develops a second cancer? What about the stress associated with the fear of losing the second breast? How does one detect cancer in the second breast or manage the remaining breast? The proposition of recalcitrant cancer in the remaining unaffected breast raises many difficult questions.

A study done many years ago showed that the opposite breast was the most common site for developing a second cancer and that there was a tissue specificity when it developed.[129]

This may be due to the fact that when breast cancer is diagnosed early it has a good prognosis. Many patients live for 10, 15, or 20 years, which provides ample time for the woman to develop a second primary cancer.

The recent development and acceptance of mammography has dramatically increased the detection of early breast cancers that can't be felt. Our diagnostic methods have taken a giant step with mammography, but we now have to improve our treatment methods to increase women's survival rates. A recent study done in Denmark,[130] showed that for a woman diagnosed with breast cancer at 45 years of age or younger, the probability of developing a contralateral breast cancer is 25 percent, if she lives to age 75. In other words, one in four women will develop a second cancer if they live long enough.

Because of this high incidence of second cancers developing, many breast cancer specialists[131,132,133] have suggested that a biopsy of the opposite breast be done routinely after the first breast cancer is discovered. Fisher and others,[134,135] however, believe that a contralateral breast biopsy has no value and that the patient can be followed adequately by frequent office visits and mammography.

Contralateral breast biopsy findings are interesting and have presented questions about how the patient should be treated, as pre-invasive and invasive cancers have been found in the second breast. The discovery of second cancers through contralateral breast biopsy has varied—2 percent in the Mayo Clinic series[136] to 12.5 percent in the series reported by Urban[131] and the more recent report by Frachia.[137] Most of the cases detected by Urban were either non–infiltrating cancers or in situ cancers.

When a second cancer is discovered by breast self-examination, the lesions are usually larger. Most are infiltrating cancers that have spread to the axillary lymph nodes. If the lesion found in the second breast is an in situ lobular carcinoma, the management is quite controversial and diametrically opposed views prevail as to proper treatment. Some suggest conservative management such as close observation, while others suggest a total mastectomy. Some women will insist that their breasts be preserved and will opt for lumpectomy (axillary dissection followed by radiation). Others will insist that all of their breast tissue be removed by bilateral mastectomies and others will insist on immediate reconstruction with silicone implants. Unfortunately most of these new techniques don't have sufficient data to back the defense of their use. The best advice I can offer is that each case has to be individualized and the wishes of the patient have to be considered and respected in the final decision.

The five-year survival rates are best if the bilateral breast cancers are picked up at the same time (synchronously).[138] This seems to support the practice of contralateral breast biopsies. There are others who feel that it is sufficient to follow breast cancer patients with careful physical and mammographic examination rather than contralateral biopsies or mastectomies.[138] The most important factor in regard to survival when a cancer develops in the opposite breast is whether the axillary glands are involved. If they are, the survival rate drops precipitously. Today, with aggressive chemotherapy, that survival rate may improve, and other methods such as enhanced immunotherapy may be on the horizon.

INCIDENCE AND RISK FACTORS

If a woman has a breast cancer, her overall risk of developing a contralateral second breast cancer (synchronous or metachronous) varies from 2.8 percent to 21 percent depending on what study you read and whether a hospital-based or population-based study was done.[139,140,138]

A population-based study[130] was completed in 1980 in Denmark on over 56,000 women from 1943 to 1980. It found that the overall relative risk of invasive cancer in the opposite breast following a first primary breast cancer to be 2.8 percent. Unfortunately, the statistics in this study include cases that pre-date mammography (1958–1962) and are probably not valid today. Recent studies done by Egan[141] at Emory University (1976) show that detection of synchronous primary breast cancers is two to seven times greater with the extensive use of mammography. It is quite evident that as radiologists become more proficient in detecting breast cancer with mammography, more and more synchronous bilateral breast cancer cases will be picked up.

There are certain known risk factors to developing a cancer in the opposite breast: the age of the patient at the time of the onset is one. Patients younger than 50 seem to have a greater risk than older patients.[142,143]

Another suggested risk factor is radiation itself. Many studies have suggested that there is a cancer-causing effect of radiation to the breast, and though the risk is greatest for younger age groups, it is present for women of all ages. When a woman has x-ray therapy after surgery for primary cancer, the tissues adjacent to the treated area (the opposite breast) receive a sufficient scatter of radiation to place the second breast at increased risk to develop cancer.

Hankey[144] and others[145] were the first to suggest that radiation treatment might be a risk factor for the development of a second breast cancer. Other researchers[140] were unable to confirm this.

Mammography is now picking up many nonpalpable cancers of the breast and more and more women are opting for limited surgery followed by radiation therapy to preserve their breasts. If there is an added risk to the opposite breast by this treatment, statistically it will almost certainly show up in the future. Land and others[146] have shown that it usually takes five to fifteen years between exposure and development of breast cancer. In my experience it sometimes takes longer. In an excellent study done at the Connecticut Tumor Registry,[143] it was reported that women who received initial radiotherapy, compared with those who did not, were at a slightly higher risk of developing a cancer in the opposite breast.

SUMMARY

Breast cancer, one of the most frequent cancers found in women, will affect one in nine women. With the advancement of mammography during the past 25 years, the detection of breast cancer has improved dramatically, and tumors that can't be felt are being detected. When the presence of more small tumors is picked up, it means that treatment methods can be more conservative, and that survival rates should improve. It also means that since more women are living longer, they can develop a cancer in the opposite breast. If a woman does develop a breast cancer before the age of 45 years, she has a 25 percent chance of developing a contralateral breast cancer if she lives to the age of 75 (one in four).[130] Since radiation therapy is being used more frequently following lumpectomy, the role of radiation in the development of cancer in the opposite breast can only be evaluated in a well-designed study of long-term survivors.

QUESTIONS

Q. What is meant by a synchronous contralateral breast cancer?

A. It means that cancers in both breasts are detected at the same time.

Q. What is meant by a metachronous contralateral breast cancer?

A. It means that the contralateral breast cancer occurs in the opposite breast after one year. There are some who feel that most second cancers, although clinically metachronous, are probably biologically synchronous.

Q. Does radiation therapy put the patient at increased risk to get a cancer in her opposite breast?

A. A definitive yes or no can't be given yet to that question. It depends somewhat on how the radiation therapy is given and whether it is monitored properly. We do know that radiation has an effect on the immune system. I feel that the patient is at a slightly increased risk to get a second primary cancer.

Q. Do you think we will be discovering more bilateral breast cancers in the future?

A. Yes. With better monitoring devices such as mammography, ultrasound, and magnification techniques, we will see more synchronous and metachronous contralateral breast cancers.

Q. Which breast cancer has the greatest effect on survival rates—the first or second breast cancer?

A. Usually the size of the second primary breast cancer is smaller than the first and is usually detected by mammography. Based on size alone, the second cancer should have a better prognosis.

Q. Do we know the best way to treat bilateral synchronous breast cancer?

A. That's a hard question to answer because there are so many variables. Cancer in the opposite breast can be a small, minimal cancer or a larger, infiltrating cancer. Or there can be two minimal cancers or two infiltrating ductal cancers. The treatment methods vary and some are still controversial, but there is no standardized treatment for the condition at the present time.

17

Are Hormones Really to Blame?

Estrogens are female hormones produced mainly by the ovaries. They are largely responsible for the changes that take place in young girls at puberty. By their direct action they cause the development of the breasts through the formation of breast ductal growth. Estrogens also cause the growth and development of the vagina, uterus, and fallopian tubes. During a normal menstrual cycle, they stimulate the breasts to enlarge and become fuller. Estrogens are also made in the placenta and adrenal glands and can be manufactured by the liver and skeletal muscle when acting with other steroid hormone precursors.

In the course of a woman's life, as menopause approaches, she experiences a natural decrease in estrogen production. As the amount of estrogens decrease in the blood some women develop classical symptoms related to menopause; however, many do not. The majority of women go through menopause without any problems. Some women develop vasomotor symptoms such as hot flashes. Symptoms of atrophic vaginitis (dryness and pain during intercourse) can develop and interfere with a woman's normal lifestyle. Osteoporosis (the washing out of calcium in bones) is known to occur in a small percentage of postmenopausal women.

125

When menopausal symptoms develop, some doctors will routinely put them on replacement therapy (estrogens). Estrogen, touted as the "feminine forever" drug, was one of the most frequently prescribed drugs of the early 1970's. Millions of menopausal women received estrogen, hoping to restore their hormonal balance and relieve the distress that sometimes accompanies the change of life.

The estrogen replacement therapy worked, but then a series of studies[147,148] found that women taking the drug for prolonged periods (more than two years) had four to eight times greater chance of developing breast cancer than women who did not receive the hormone. They were also at risk for endometrial cancer. For many menopausal women it was a fearful discovery: estrogen's risks suddenly appeared greater than any benefits. When this adverse, alarming fact became known to the public, the drug manufacturers added progestin to help neutralize the estrogen effect and hopefully decrease the risk of cancer. The media have reported that the risk of cancer has been lessened, but it is still too early to tell if this is true.

It has been difficult to evaluate the effects of estrogen and progestin on the breast during and after menopause. Combination therapy has been widely used in the 1980's and only recently have research studies[149] been published concerning it. Researchers from the National Cancer Institute and the University Hospital in Upsala, Sweden, studied over 23,000 women over 35 who used non-contraceptive estrogen. Their risk of breast cancer increased 10 percent by taking estrogen prescribed for menopausal symptoms (that is, non-contraceptive estrogen) and the risk increased with duration of use. And combination therapy with progestin (the new pill) *increased* the risk of breast cancer.

There are other adverse effects from excessive use of estrogens during menopause. Indiscriminate hormone replacement with high doses of estrogen has been shown in experimental research to promote tissue growth in both animal and human breasts.[150,151] Other studies have linked high estrogen levels in women in high-risk groups to development of cancer of the endometrium of the uterus.[152,153,154,155]

ESTROGENS AND MENOPAUSE

The use of estrogens during menopause and their effect on breast tissue has been a matter of controversy in medical circles for years. The possibility of increased risk has been noted by the National Institute of Health and no one knows what the long-term effects will be. But this much seems evident: the longer you take estrogen, the greater the risk.

Estrogen receptors in the majority of breast tumors and the clinical response to hormonal therapy—especially estrogen blocking agents, such as Tamoxifen—suggests that there is no doubt about the influence of hormones on the progression of breast cancer. This is why women and physicians should take a much closer look at what for years has been an accepted practice.

Today, more than seven million women past menopause are taking estrogen supplements or the new combination pill containing estrogen and progestin. Why? Aside from relieving some menopausal symptoms, these women erroneously believe that estrogen will keep them looking young, prevent their breasts from sagging, and prolong their lives. There is no evidence that estrogen will do any of these things. There is, however, firm evidence that prolonged use of estrogen *will* increase the risk of breast cancer. [156,157,158]

Doctors who routinely prescribe estrogen supplements are not allowing the body's natural physiological mechanisms to adapt to the changes occurring. Menopause is not a single event but a process that takes place over about 15 years, from about the age of 40 to 60.

The first missed menstrual period is definitely not a signal of menopause. So, forget whatever you may have heard about the onset of "the change" and seek a second opinion before starting estrogen therapy. More likely than not, once menopause begins, the only change you will notice is one for the better.

Only 10 to 15 percent of menopausal women really need treatment. But many can benefit from alternative therapies. For example, to relieve vaginal dryness you can use a water-soluble lubricant during intercourse. Brittle bones (osteoporosis) will respond to a diet high in calcium and protein and vigorous exercise can help maintain bone strength. The exact role of estrogens in preventing osteoporosis is still controversial.

With all that has been written about the problems of menopause, we sometimes tend to forget that the vast majority of women pass through this stage of life without a major problem and require no treatment or medication. For those who do experience problems, there are many safe alternatives to estrogen. Don't hesitate to discuss alternatives with your gynecologist or family doctor. Even when the doctor prescribes estrogens (typically after induced menopause or hysterectomy) you should be concerned about the dosage and length of treatment. Ask your doctor to explain why he is prescribing estrogens.

QUESTIONS

Q. What should a woman do if she develops hot flashes at the menopause and has difficulty tolerating them?

A. First, she should see her physician. There are many methods other than estrogens that aid in controlling hot flashes. Tranquilizers can be used. Emotional support by the physician at this time is helpful, too. If it is necessary to use estrogens, only minimal doses should be taken and close follow-up by the physician will ensure that adverse side effects do not occur.

Q. How long should a woman continue to take estrogens?

A. Each case is different, but there has to be a cutoff time. I recently saw an 81–year-old patient with breast cancer who was still taking estrogens and had not seen her gynecologist for 15 years. Unmonitored, continuous estrogen supplements like this can be really hazardous.

Q. Are there some women who should not be given estrogen supplements?

A. Yes. Estrogen supplements should not be used by women who have severe liver disease (alcoholics and cirrhotics), or those with blood clotting disorders or severe heart disease. Estrogen is detoxified mainly in the liver and if the liver is damaged, retention of excessive estrogens occurs. A small amount of estrogen is excreted in the bile and is reabsorbed by the intestines. The liver is involved in blood clotting mechanisms and the indiscriminate use of estrogens can be hazardous to that function, too.

Q. Some women seem to breeze through menopause with few symptoms and others seem to have difficulty with severe hot flashes. Why is that?

A. Vasomotor flushes or sweats are poorly understood symptoms and not all women experience them. These eventually subside without treatment.

Q. What should you do if you feel that you absolutely need estrogen therapy?

A. To reduce the risk of getting cancer, estrogen therapy, if given at all, should be given in conjunction with progestins and should be the lowest dosage possible. However, there is some recent evidence that suggests the addition of progestin may not protect against breast cancer. Consult your doctor. In those women who are in a high-risk group for breast cancer, hormone therapy should not be given at all if the woman is post-menopausal. It also should not be given to women who have cancer of the reproductive organs.

Q. *What if a woman has a hysterectomy and oophorectomy (ovary removal) early in life and needs estrogen replacement therapy?*

A. Women who have hysterectomies early in life and are in a high-risk group for breast cancer should be watched very carefully if they are on replacement estrogen therapy. The level of estrogens should be minimal and combined with progestins.

Q. *If a woman has a hysterectomy and oophorectomy will she be protected from breast cancer?*

A. Seventeen percent of my breast cancer patients had hysterectomies and oophorectomies and took replacement therapy. It's obvious it did not protect these women from getting breast cancer.

Q. *How does a doctor advise a patient whether or not she should take estrogens, particularly since the risk factors may outweigh the benefits?*

A. The decision has to be made by the patient and the doctor. It definitely has to be individualized. The woman must be absolutely sure that she is getting accurate information. It's a personal decision in which the doctor must express an opinion about the current understanding of the treatment's effectiveness at the time of the decision. To make this choice intelligently, the woman must be given all the information available about the positive and negative effects of the use of estrogens. It should also be remembered that some patients require estrogens for specific medical reasons outside of coping with menopause.

THE BIRTH CONTROL PILL

The recent anniversary of the birth control pill has been embraced by its manufacturers as an occasion to mount a publicity campaign to tell women the Pill is safer than ever. How much of this hoopla is hype? The sensitive response should be healthy skepticism. For while the Pill remains unsurpassed for convenience and effectiveness, the question of its safety persists.

In fact, the question most asked about the birth control pill is the same one posed years ago: "Does the Pill cause cancer?" The answer to that is still not a clear yes or no but a number of studies begin to give us some definitive answers. One of these, done in Los Angeles by a British doctor, Malcolm C. Pike,[159] did show an increased rate of breast cancer in young women taking birth control pills. However, since most of the women studied until now have been in their 50's (when the Pill contained large amounts of estrogen) the cause-and-effect relationship to breast cancer is not clear-cut. A controversy still exists as to whether the birth control pill increases or decreases the risk of breast cancer, and research in this area is extremely difficult because so many variables have been introduced.

During the past 25 years there has been a change in the chemical make-up and potency of the Pill. The content of both the estrogen and pro-gestogen steroids in the Pill have decreased. In 1964, 92 percent of the Pills marketed contained more than 50 mg of estrogen. By 1983 only 9 percent of the Pills prescribed had more than 50 mg of estrogen and 52 percent had less than 50 mg of progestogen.[159,160]

Two recent studies add coals to the fire of controversy. Research conducted by Oxford University and the Institute of Cancer Research found that young women who take the birth control pill for more than four years run a significantly greater risk of developing breast cancer than those who use other methods of contraception. The study, published in the May issue of *Lancet* 1989,[161] showed that the risk of breast cancer among women under age 36 was increased 74 percent by long-term use (eight years or more) of oral contraceptives. For research purposes the British system of documenting medical history is very accurate since they have a national health care system—English citizens have a perma-nent lifelong medical record.

Another important recent study[162] of the birth control pill was done by Dr. Hakar Olson from the University Hospital in Lund, Sweden (1989). The birth control pill was widely used there by teenagers after its intro-duction in the 1960's, and the incidence of breast cancer among women under age 40 has risen in Sweden since its advent. Some researchers feel that the Swedish study suggests that the birth control pill is linked to early, premenopausal breast cancer.

Another study,[163] conducted at Harvard University (a ten-year study of 118,273 women), found that middle-aged women who waited to take the birth control pill until after their mid-twenties had no unusual risk of breast cancer. Comparison of the Harvard Study with the Swedish (Uni-versity Hospital of Lund) and Oxford University studies suggest there is a conflict. It's possible that the Pill's effects are different in very young women, since the Harvard study was done in women over 25 years of age. The Harvard study also substantiated the Oxford study, by indicating there was a 50 percent increase in the risk of breast cancer among women who took the pill after age 40.

The Pill works by altering the body's hormonal balance so the ovaries do not produce the eggs necessary for fertilization. There is also a thickening of the mucous lining of the uterus that prevents the sperm from fertilizing any egg that is produced. The latter is caused by progestin (a form of progesterone), present in both the combined and so-called "mini" pills.

Taking the Pill also increases the rate of cell division in the lobules of the breast, which is what happens in the growth of a cancerous tumor.[164] Studies have shown that progesterone can cause breast hyperplasia (considered a precancerous condition) and lobular carcinomas when taken in large doses or for extended periods of time.[165] This is particularly true for first-generation birth control pills that women began taking in the 1960's, which contained more estrogen.

There is also evidence that women who have never had children are at greater risk of developing breast cancer. Their breasts are being stimulated by estrogen longer than those women who become pregnant. The longer a woman waits to have her first baby, the less opportunity there is for the natural protective effect of pregnancy and lactation.[166] What this means is that young women who take the Pill and have never been pregnant lack an adequate response to the progesterone (the antagonist to estrogen in the Pill). Such women will, in effect, be exposing their breasts to unopposed estrogen and will be at increased risk for developing breast cancer.[167] The following case history demonstrates this effect on the body's normal defense mechanisms.

A patient of mine, a young woman 24 years old, was examined and a lump was found in her right breast which mammograms confirmed as cancerous. She had been taking the Pill for five years beginning at age 17, and then stopped, hoping to get pregnant. The medications she then received to regain her normal menstrual cycle contained high doses of estrogen and progestin. She did not regain a normal menstrual cycle, the lump persisted, and a biopsy was done.

The biopsy revealed an invasive ductal cancer of the breast and nipple and she was admitted to the hospital for further diagnostic testing. A liver scan showed extensive spread of the cancer to her liver. Intensive medical oncologic treatment with chemotherapy was started. However, because of the advanced stage of her breast cancer, the woman died four months after her initial biopsy. This case demonstrates what can happen to a young woman if her body cannot react properly to an exogenous alteration in her hormonal status.

Complications of the Birth Control Pill

Many adverse side effects developed from the use of the early Pill; strokes, heart attacks, severe migraine headaches, phlebitis, diabetes, and cancer. Most were related to either the estrogen or progestin content in the pill and specific research documented these problems.

Vascular changes occur and are probably related to the progestin dose in the Pill. If progestogens are added to the Pill, there also seems to be an added coronary risk. Estrogens seem to decrease this risk. The media have recently suggested that the Pill can be safely used in the older age group. Don't believe this until more accurate research has been done.

BIOPSY AND BENIGN BREAST DISEASE

If the apparent link between the Pill and breast cancer is confirmed, it will be particularly bad news for women with benign breast disease or fibrocystic disease—a condition that may cause discomfort but in no way threatens a woman's life. The Pill has been shown to prevent benign breast disease and to shrink or eliminate breast cysts around the time of ovulation by suppressing the normal hormonal cycle that causes the cysts to appear.[168,169] This condition is most common in younger women but should not indicate a biopsy is necessary—even in those women who are not on the Pill.

In fact, the incidence of biopsies for benign breast disease has greatly decreased in recent years with the advent of imaging techniques (mammography) and more frequent breast self-examination. Biopsies are also more meaningful and have helped to eliminate needless surgery. There's really no reason for a woman with fibrocystic breast disease (discussed in Chapter 7) to be unduly concerned that she will get breast cancer.

SUMMARY

Is the Pill safer than it was, because the estrogen dosage has been substantially reduced and progestin has been added? Or is there an added risk, as some researchers suggest? The Pill may benefit some users but there is still some controversy about its safety. There is little doubt about the link between estrogen and breast cancer, especially in women who take the Pill for long periods of time. The long-term results of the use of oral contraceptives will take many more years to evaluate. The study of exposure to diethylstilbestrol during pregnancy in the 1950's showed a doubling of breast cancer risk, but not until 22 years later. Also, it is a well known fact that the age at which a woman starts menstruating affects her risk of getting breast cancer 25 or more years later. Until more studies are done, it's up to each woman to reach her own decision based on the evidence. She should also consult her doctor.

QUESTIONS

Q. What if you want to take the Pill?
A. Don't take it if you smoke or are over 35 years of age. In any case, watch carefully for any danger signals: blood clots, pain in the abdomen, numbness in the arm, or growths in the breast.

Q. Are there any benefits to taking the Pill?
A. Yes. Aside from preventing pregnancy and benign breast disease, the Pill has been shown to lower the incidence of pelvic inflammatory disease (PID), which is a common cause of infertility. It has also reduced the rate of iron-deficiency anemia caused by long menstrual periods and excessive blood loss.

Q. Can taking the Pill affect any medical tests?
A. Yes. Thyroid function tests can be affected, as can blood glucose and plasma insulin tests.

Q. Should women taking the Pill still have other tests done?
A. Definite monthly breast self-examination is a must as well as an annual check-up. Routine Pap smears should also be done and the abdomen palpated (for evidence of liver enlargement).

Q. Did any of your breast cancer patients take the Pill?
A. Yes. Seventeen percent of my patients who developed breast cancer were on the birth control pill. Many of these women took the Pill when it contained high doses of estrogen. This suggests that the early birth control pill does not protect you from getting breast cancer.

Q. Since progestin was added to the birth control pill in the early 1980's, have any of your patients on the new Pill gotten breast cancer?
A. The answer is yes.

Q. *Do you feel the birth control pill causes cancer?*

A. I don't think anybody can answer that question. I worry about it. I have tried to point out some of the beneficial and harmful effects of the Pill. There is no doubt the Pill has been improved but all the facts are still not in. One of the biggest problems is to try and define those women who would be at increased risk if they take the Pill. Recent genetic research studies may give insight into how to solve this problem, and I believe it can be solved in the future. There is no doubt that some women are hurt by the Pill, but it may take many years and a few generations to determine its long-term effects. The birth control pill has some good effects for some patients and some bad effects for others. It's the woman's choice if she wishes to take that unknown risk.

18

Brittle Bones After Menopause

"Damned if you do, damned if you don't." This statement applies to estrogen-replacement therapy as a universal remedy for postmenopausal women. If you take estrogens, you are less likely to develop bone loss associated with menopause and aging. (It does not totally prevent osteoporosis.) However, you are possibly at greater risk for breast cancer or endometrial cancer if you take replacement estrogens.

During a woman's life her ovarian function diminishes and at approximately 51 years (average) she has her last episode of uterine bleeding, indicating the onset of menopause. Hormonal changes at menopause bring on several physiological changes in a woman's body; these may be vasomotor changes (hot flashes) that persist for one to five years, and numerous somatic complaints such as anxiety, depression, headaches, and irritability. Atrophy of the reproductive organs and lower urinary tracts as well as increased susceptibility to infection and inflammation can also occur. Vaginal dryness, burning, itching, and pain during intercourse are also quite common.

There are now approximately 40 million women in the United States who are either approaching menopause or are in it. Not all women

135

develop symptoms associated with "the change of life." Some women breeze right through it and require no medication; others take a long time to adapt to the loss of estrogens.

Unfortunately, most obstetricians and gynecologists routinely prescribe estrogens during menopause when a woman complains about vague symptoms. Some are prescribing the new drugs that have added progestin, hoping to prevent the risk of breast cancer and endometrial cancer. But prescribing hormone drugs is a tremendous expense and has to be monitored to determine its usefulness. It sometimes takes extensive research over twenty-five years to determine beneficial or harmful effects of drugs.

As a woman ages, one of the most important changes that occurs at menopause is osteoporosis. Women's bones become soft and demineralized; a calcium imbalance develops and bone resorption takes place. Being a couch potato and immobile contributes to washing out of the bones. Women who exercise regularly and maintain a vigorous level of activity have healthy bones longer despite the aging process.

As a result of calcium washing out of bones, postmenopausal women often suffer vertebral compression fractures and hip fractures. It has been estimated that 20 percent of women have one or more such fractures (vertebral, wrist, or proximal femur) by the age of 65.[170] Since the life expectancy of women in this country is 79 years, approximately 40 percent will suffer fractures after the age of 65 years. Over six million people in the United States have some form of osteoporosis, and yet it usually does not occur in men until after 60 years of age.

Many doctors feel that osteoporosis is a serious health hazard linked directly to menopause. They also feel that giving estrogen replacement therapy to the postmenopausal female, in most cases, will prevent the onset of "brittle bones." Some doctors throw up their hands when they are confronted with the "brittle bones" problem—they say they don't know how to treat or prevent it.

Reduction in bone mass after menopause is not completely related to the loss of estrogens, although it would be nice from a medical standpoint if it were. Although many women demonstrate considerable bone loss after menopause, the majority will not experience symptomatic osteoporosis. Yet doctors often prescribe estrogen to forestall osteoporosis, even though the mechanism of the action of estrogen replacement therapy is still elusive and unknown. The only known effect of estrogen replacement therapy in the treatment of osteoporosis is that it inhibits bone resorption.

Many physiological effects of the aging process are interrelated. Cardiac, lung, kidney, endocrine, and gastrointestinal disease may contribute to the etiology of osteoporosis. Critical organs and glands do not function as well when we get older, and the interrelationship and mechanisms involved in osteoporosis may well be linked to the function of other organs and processes.

Research scientists feel the role of estrogen replacement therapy in the aging process needs further clarification and should not be prescribed as a matter of course. Hormonal replacement therapy carries many risks and requires medical supervision. Be sure that you're fully informed and ask your gynecologist about complications that can develop with the use of estrogens. Some concerns to raise with him or her are: endometrial cancer, breast cancer, hypertension, hyperlipidemia, and gallbladder disease.

We do know that there are many different factors that play roles in keeping a woman's bones healthy after menopause. Adequate calcium intake, estrogens, physical activity (exercise), vitamin D (sunlight), steroids (androgens), calcitonin, parathyroid hormones, and fluorides are just a few necessities.

DIET

A lifetime of adequate calcium intake is one of the best ways to avoid osteoporosis. In order to utilize dietary calcium intake an adequate supply of vitamin D is important. This can be obtained either in the diet or by skin exposure to sunlight. In countries with limited sunlight or where the population typically dresses so that minimal sunlight exposure occurs, circulating levels of vitamin D are low and this leads to less bone-mass formation.

Physiologically, vitamin D serves to maintain a normal serum calcium concentration in the bloodstream and maintains a proper calcium transport system in the intestines. The vitamin D endocrine system is an important calcium stabilizer.

Americans generally seem to get enough sunlight and vitamin D deficiency is not a problem. It is extremely important for menopausal women to have an adequate daily calcium intake. Good sources of calcium are milk, nuts, wheat flour breads, yogurt, Swiss and cheddar cheese, molasses, and vegetables high in calcium such as kidney beans, broccoli, and spinach. Women on diets can take equivalent calcium tablets if they so desire. The average calcium intake should be 1,500 mg per day.

EXERCISE

Active growing children on healthy diets influence their skeletal mass by making stringent demands on their bones. Athletes, cross-country runners, and weight lifters all have more bone mass than the average person. But even if you're not an athlete, adequate calcium intake is necessary for exercise to have an affect on bone mass.

Our space program has dramatically demonstrated that loss of bone mass occurs rapidly with both lack of exercise and the effect of gravity on our ambulation. The reduced physical activity and weightlessness in space can be tolerated for just so long.

People who are injured and are bedridden for long periods of time lose bone mass too. This means that daily exercise is critical in maintaining normal skeletal bone. Brisk walking, bicycle riding, and participating in sports that place demands on your body will help maintain healthy bone mass.

SEX HORMONES

Here is a brief summation of what we do and do not know about the influence of sex hormones on bone mass: Women who have children have a higher bone mass than those who do not; frequency of lactation is associated with increased bone mass; hormones play a role in maintaining a normal healthy bone mass but their exact action is unknown; women who take oral contraceptives, which contain hormones, seem to increase their bone mass density.

Obesity too seems to play a role in increased hormone production. It's ironic that obesity offers protection against getting brittle bones and fractures, yet has been identified as a risk factor for breast cancer. The ingestion of animal fats (triglycerides) and the development of obesity puts women at added risk for breast cancer, as obese women have greater body weight, causing increased peripheral estrogen production. The increased estrogen may, however, protect them against osteoporosis. To complicate the problem further, it's known that vegetarians are at low risk for osteoporosis and most vegetarians are thin with low body weight. Admittedly, the scenario of interrelationships of osteoporosis and hormones, age, fitness, and nutrition is a complex and cluttered one.

Yet there is one more subtlety to consider. When women became afraid to take estrogens at menopause because of the added risk for breast cancer, drug manufacturers in the early 1980's added progestin as an antagonist to estrogens. However, recent studies show the addition of progestin does not remove the risk for breast cancer and endometrial cancer but may actually *add* to the risks.

SUMMARY

The insidious loss of bone mass, seen primarily in the vertebrae, wrist, and hips of postmenopausal women has resulted in a female segment of the population that must endure old age with "brittle bones." This fact, coupled with the extended life expectancy of women, has made medical care for this problem costly. As this cost now approaches four billion dollars a year, no one factor has been identified as the primary cause. Diets deficient in calcium; lack of vitamin D, estrogen deprivation, and so forth are understood to be contributing causes of osteoporosis, but all the facts are not known and additional research is needed.

QUESTIONS

Q. *At the time of menopause, should a woman be thin or fat if she wants to avoid getting osteoporosis?*

A. Obese women produce more estrogen than thin women. Therefore, thin women are at greater risk for fractures. Vegetarians, however, are usually thin and are less apt to get "brittle bones." Maintaining a normal healthy weight for your age should be the objective.

Q. *Do black or white women have more osteoporotic fractures?*

A. Black women have fewer fractures because they have a higher bone mass, greater bone density, and greater density in their vertebral bones.

Q. *Does smoking have anything to do with brittle bones (osteoporosis)?*

A. Most studies show that smoking is associated with reduced bone mass as well as increased risk of vertebral and hip fractures. This may have something to do with the hepatic metabolism of estrogen. Most smokers have less adipose tissue and therefore less circulating estrogen.

Q. *Are there any recent advances in technology for evaluating bone mass and predicting osteoporosis?*

A. X-ray techniques using CT scan (Computerized Axial Tomography) are helpful in evaluating and monitoring osteoporosis. There still isn't a good method for screening large populations.

Q. *Is exercise important to maintain healthy bones?*

A. It's clear that daily vigorous physical activity is important in maintaining good bone mass and skeletal strength.

Q. *How much calcium should a postmenopausal woman take daily?*

A. At least 1,500 mg per day. Vitamin D should also be taken to assist in calcium absorption.

Q. *If a woman frequently drinks beverages which contain caffeine, such as coffee or cola, does it alter her calcium intake after menopause?*

A. Yes. Caffeine causes increased excretion of calcium in the urine, which means that the daily calcium intake has to be increased.

Q. *In some sections of the country, water purifiers are used to make water drinkable. Could this play a possible role in osteoporosis?*

A. Yes. Most reservoir water supplies have added fluorides. Studies show that osteoporosis is lower in areas with high fluoride levels in the drinking water, and some water purifiers eliminate the fluorides.

Q. *Is there anything new in the treatment regimen of osteoporosis to reduce the incidence of bone fractures?*

A. Yes. A recent research article in the *New England Journal of Medicine*[171] reported that women treated for two years with etidronate disodium and calcium had fewer fractures of the spine than women who did not take the drug. The drug did not prevent fractures in all the women treated, however.

Q. *Does fluoride treatment decrease the fracture rate in postmenopausal women with osteoporosis?*

A. Fluoride therapy increases cancellous bone but decreases cortical bone mineral density and increases skeletal fragility. In other words, fluoride calcium regimens are not effective treatment to prevent osteoporotic fractures.[172]

19

Breast Reconstruction After Mastectomy

According to a survey conducted by the American Society of Plastic and Reconstructive Surgeons, approximately 34,200 breast reconstructions were done in 1988 in the United States, an increase from an estimated 20,000 in 1981.

More than one million American women have undergone augmentation mammoplasty since the development of modern silicone-gel–filled prostheses, introduced in the early 1960's. Each year, one hundred thousand women have breast augmentation for reconstruction following mastectomy, or for reconstruction following the atrophy of pregnancy, and to enlarge small breasts. This number is increasing every year. Ten percent of women who have undergone augmentation mammoplasty have already, or can expect to develop, breast cancer.[173] In some areas of the country, women at high risk of developing breast cancer have had bilateral subcutaneous mastectomies and reconstruction with the hope of preventing it.

Why has there been such a tremendous increase in recent years in cosmetic breast surgery? There are many reasons. The technique of replacing the mound of the breast has improved immensely. A patient can

141

now select the size of the silicone implant she wants—it can be sized to match the remaining breast, or with expandable silicone implants the size can be varied relatively easily by injecting saline into the plastic bag.

The cosmetic defect created by mastectomy for treating cancer has been unacceptable to most women—many women do not like using the replaceable prosthesis even though it, too, has recently been improved.

Artists, for centuries, have considered the female form to be the ultimate expression of beauty, and attempts to duplicate it in painting or sculpture are among our most prized possessions. Women, like men, pride themselves on the appearance of their body. They join exercise clubs, aerobic classes, and often make great sacrifices and diet regularly to maintain an attractive figure.

Nobody can comprehend the tremendous psychological trauma that occurs when a woman is told she must lose a breast. When this happens, the most common feeling is that of being "half a woman" and unattractive to a male partner. One way women attempt to cope with this real or imagined fear is to seek breast reconstruction. Sometimes the result can turn a woman's life around and make her feel like a new person.

Breast cancer surgeons working with plastic surgeons have recognized the need to help these women who have had a mastectomy. During the past decade, numerous sophisticated plastic procedures have been devised to replace the mound in the breast so a woman can feel complete again and resume a normal lifestyle.

The different reconstructive procedures developed by the plastic surgeons are innovative and quite imaginative. The object is to match the size and shape of the remaining breast as closely as possible, though sometimes the remaining breast has to have a mastopexy to alter its shape in relation to the breast with the silicone implant.

The method for reconstruction depends on several factors. Not all women have the same size breasts—some breasts are large, others are small. In some cases the chest wall muscles (pectoral) have not been preserved or are damaged. Some women have had radiation therapy and the surface tissues have been damaged and have to be replaced. Then, too, not all cancer surgeons are the same—the incision may be placed in different areas. The size of the tumor (cancer) may have been small or large and greater amounts of skin may have been sacrificed. In other words, the extent of the mastectomy surgery can be radical (radical mastectomy) or moderate (modified mastectomy or simple mastectomy).

Since most patients do not know or understand plastic procedures, it is of paramount importance that an open, honest discussion of the various methods be presented to the patient so that there can be complete informed consent. Some women will request to see pictures of the reconstructive methods used by the plastic surgeon—"before-and-after" pictures. They might ask the question, "How many breast reconstructive procedures have you done following mastectomy?" Most plastic surgeons will show only their good results so it might be a good idea to ask about possible complications: Can you get an infection? Does the silicone implant leak? Does the implant ever have to be replaced? What are the chances of getting recurrent cancer after implant surgery?[173] Don't be afraid to ask questions *before* the reconstructive procedure!

There is also the question of whether reconstructive surgery can produce the desired psychological confidence the patient seeks. This is a matter of no small concern among cancer specialists and plastic surgeons who must treat the breast cancer patient in both body and spirit. They must attempt to answer her questions and determine the reasons behind them. How will it look? Will the scars go away? What about the nipple? Will it look like a real nipple? What if the cancer comes back? If a silicone implant is put into the defect, will it be harder to detect a recurrence? Does the implant prevent early detection? The woman who desires breast reconstruction has to face all these questions straight on.

HOW PATIENTS ARE SELECTED

Breast reconstruction isn't new. What is new is that there's now an easier method to replace the breast mound—the silicone implant. Surgeons are doing fewer disfiguring radical mastectomies, so plastic surgery is possible in more cases. Chest wall muscles are not being sacrificed. However, such surgery—indeed any further hospitalization—is not for every woman. Those who have already endured the trauma of cancer, mastectomy, and perhaps radiation therapy may opt to forego reconstruction.

In my opinion, breast reconstruction works best for the woman who has no doubt that it is what she wants. Since some health insurance plans, unfortunately, define any plastic surgery as "elective" or "cosmetic" a woman may need to pay the entire hospital and surgical cost herself. Age need not preclude such an operation, however. Too often the attitude of both doctors and family has been, "Why do you want reconstruction?

You should be happy just to be alive." My own experience is any woman who wishes reconstruction, and who is suitable for it, should have it.

It has been said that a woman's apparent physiological age is more important than her chronological age. I would add that a woman's psychological age, or how she creates her own lifestyle, is also vitally important. How does a person dress and look? How active is she in daily living? You can be over 70, but feel and behave like 50 or younger because you are in good physical and spiritual shape. My oldest "reconstructed" patient was 65 years old and the youngest 28.

Physicians are finally realizing what many women have been saying all along: reconstruction can add to a woman's positive feelings about herself. Some women can learn to live with one breast, others cannot. Some will not let their husbands touch them or see them undressed. They should have the option of reconstruction without having to make excuses for their choice. Some experts on aging suggest that, if a surgeon turns you down for restorative surgery just because of your age, you should get a second opinion and, if necessary, a third.

Medically speaking, the selection of patients for breast reconstruction is more clear-cut. They should have no evidence of diffuse tumor spread, bone, lung, or soft tissue metastases.

IMMEDIATE BREAST RECONSTRUCTION

There is still controversy over whether immediate breast reconstruction should be done following mastectomy. Today, approximately 25 percent of breast reconstructions are done immediately; the remaining 75 percent are done months or even years later.

Fortunately, most of these operations are performed in large centers where the procedure is done frequently. A surgical team's familiarity with the procedure can prevent serious complications that might otherwise develop.

One problem concerning immediate breast reconstruction is that it is difficult to stage the cancer during surgery—all of the resected breast tissue and glands cannot be studied to see if the tissue margins are free of cancer and whether the lymph glands are involved. Often the deep margin beneath the cancer biopsy site is also where the implant has to be placed. Multiple glands or the chest wall muscles may also be involved with the breast cancer. If this happens, the reconstruction procedure should not be done.

DELAYED BREAST RECONSTRUCTION: WHICH TYPE OF RECONSTRUCTION SHOULD BE DONE?

The majority of reconstructions (75 percent) are delayed ones. If a woman has a mastectomy and immediate reconstruction is done, there is a small risk that a calamity may occur—an infection may develop or the skin flaps may fail to heal and adhere properly. It should be noted that the trauma of the mastectomy is sometimes too much to handle, and a serious complication following it may be even more injurious to the patient. Another important fact has to be considered—the possibility of a recurrence. Most local chest wall recurrences develop within the first year of surgery.[174] However, a few can develop many years later. It's easier to watch the chest wall for recurrence if there isn't a silicone implant covering it up.

By delaying reconstruction, the patient emotionally adjusts to the loss of the breast and has time to accept the "not-so-perfect" reconstruction. It is impossible to make the breast exactly as it was before, but by waiting, the blood supply to the skin has ample time to grow in from the underlying muscle. Emotional and physical healing, for the postoperative patient, generally go hand-in-hand.

There are several different procedures that can be done, depending on the patient's condition and the skill of the surgeon. To help ensure the best results, it is wise to seek a surgeon who is board-certified by the American College of Plastic Surgery and who does frequent reconstructive breast surgery. You may ask around in your community to find out who is doing the best reconstructive surgery. You may have to seek treatment outside your local area if you live in a small community.

During the past 15 years, methods have been developed to recreate the mound of the breast with a silicone implant,[175,176] or by transferring tissue from one part of the body to another. Skin and muscle flaps with attached blood supply (myocutaneous flaps) have also been used to replace the defect created by mastectomy.[177,178,179] Skin-expander techniques and plastic prosthetic devices have likewise been improved.[180,181]

Basically, the idea is to form a pocket into which the silicone gel implant is placed (see Figure 10). If too much skin or muscle was removed in the mastectomy, a muscle-skin flap might have to be created. For the woman with a good skin-and-muscle base over the chest wall, silicone implantation and reconstruction is a one-stage procedure. Some surgeons

Figure 10
SIMPLE SILICONE IMPLANT—MOST POPULAR RECONSTRUCTION FOLLOWING MASTECTOMY

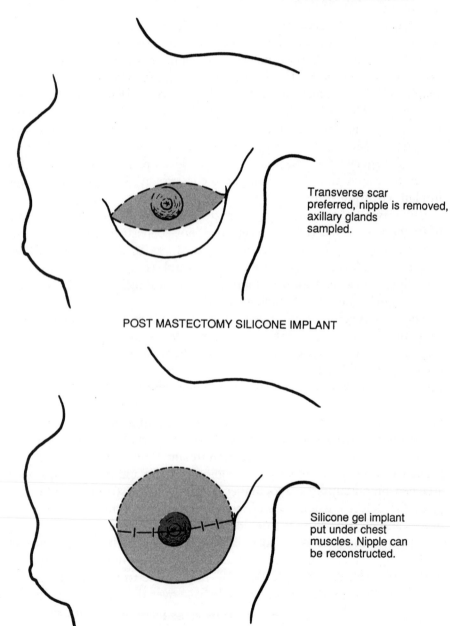

Transverse scar preferred, nipple is removed, axillary glands sampled.

POST MASTECTOMY SILICONE IMPLANT

Silicone gel implant put under chest muscles. Nipple can be reconstructed.

SIMPLEST AND MOST POPULAR RECONSTRUCTION FOLLOWING MASTECTOMY

are now doing mastectomy with a horizontal incision that follows the skin's natural tension lines and is easier to repair. The surgeon who does the mastectomy should always think about where to place the skin incision so that a better cosmetic effect will result if reconstruction is anticipated.

A small implant is used at first, so the blood supply is not hindered and the skin-and-muscle tissue is gradually stretched. If the patient desires, a larger implant can be inserted at a later date. Silicone implants are now available that can be expanded without another operation.[181] Patients who are very thin or who have had radiation therapy, which may harden the skin, are not good candidates for silicone implants and may require muscle and skin transfer procedures.

Omental tissue transfer

Another technique[182] is to use a portion of the greater omentum to furnish both tissue and blood supply to the chest wall. The greater omentum is an apron-like structure that hangs down from the greater curvature of the stomach, in front of the colon. It contains fat, lymphatic channels and lymph nodes, and is brought out through an incision in the abdomen and tunneled under the skin of the mastectomy site. It forms a soft rubbery substance and gives a soft feel to the replaced mound of the breast. Once the omentum has attached itself to the chest wall, the silicone implant is placed under the omentum (see Figure 11).

Figure 11
OMENTAL TISSUE TRANSFER RECONSTRUCTION

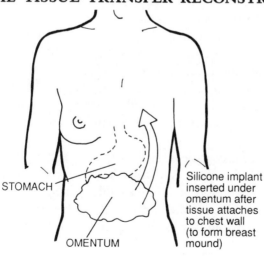

STOMACH

OMENTUM

Silicone implant
inserted under
omentum after
tissue attaches
to chest wall
(to form breast
mound)

Transverse Rectus Abdominus Muscle Flap Reconstruction (TRAM)

This plastic procedure uses the rectus muscle and skin of the lower belly with its blood supply and is transferred to the chest-wall defect (mastectomy site). A tummy tuck results from a tightening of the abdominal wall. This procedure is used when a lot of skin and muscle has been taken with the mastectomy (see Figure 12).[183,184,185]

Latissimus Dorsi Muscle Transfer[186]

In this operation, the plastic surgeon transfers a large muscle from the back, with its skin and blood supply, to the mastectomy site. A silicone implant is then placed under the new chest muscle. This technique is often used when a radical mastectomy has been done (see Figure 13).

There are also other methods of tissue transfer such as microscopic transfer of tissue with blood supply and abdominal tissue advancement techniques. When a skin-flap procedure is needed a breast can be reconstructed with fat and skin from the buttocks. The tissue for the breast reconstruction is elevated on a vascular pedicle, or support. This method can provide reconstruction without a silicone breast implant.[187]

Unfortunately, not every woman with a mastectomy qualifies for breast reconstruction for either physical or psychological reasons. Almost 50 percent of women, when first diagnosed with breast cancer, will exhibit regional glandular spread or spread to other areas of the body. About 10 percent of women with breast cancer will present with minimal cancer; that is, tumors small enough to be eligible for limited surgery (lumpectomy or quadrectomy). That percentage is increasing rapidly as more and more minimal cancers are being detected by mammography.

Reconstruction can restore a woman's cleavage so that, when clothed, she looks and feels normal again. It cannot, of course, restore the physical function of the chest muscles, but where tactility is concerned, the new silicone gel implants feel almost completely the same as a normal, healthy breast.

Radical mastectomy patients have a more difficult problem in reconstruction because the chest wall muscles have been removed with the breast tissue and therefore it is impossible to simply put a silicone gel implant under the skin of the chest wall. These patients require more extensive plastic procedures involving muscle and skin transfers.

Figure 12
TRANSVERSE RECTUS ABDOMINUS MUSCLE FLAP RECONSTRUCTION (TRAM)

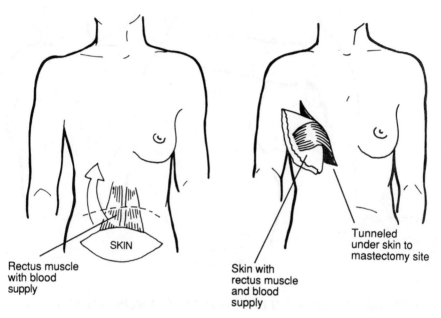

Rectus muscle
with blood
supply

SKIN

Skin with
rectus muscle
and blood
supply

Tunneled
under skin to
mastectomy site

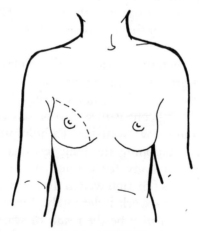

Flap sutured in place
with reconstructed nipple
(silicone implant may or
may not be used)

Figure 13
LATISSIMUS DORSI MUSCLE TRANSFER
RECONSTRUCTION

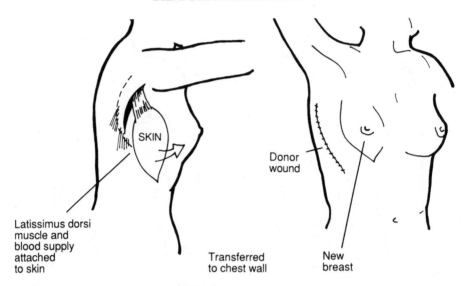

Latissimus dorsi muscle and blood supply attached to skin

SKIN

Transferred to chest wall

Donor wound

New breast

SOME PROBLEMS WITH SILICONE PROSTHESES

Many years ago, women had foreign material (such as silicone) injected with a needle and syringe into their breasts to increase their breast size or to make them appear firmer. Some of these women later developed cancer of the breast.

Today, the silicone material is placed within a plastic shell, and some of the new silicone gel prostheses have a button into which more material can be injected or removed if the woman wishes a larger or smaller sized breast. Either way, the silicone is meant to be self-contained.

Breast expanders are now available. Pathologists and other experts recently have been questioning the long-term safety of materials implanted into the human body for medical or cosmetic reasons. Most modern silicone implants function well in the breasts for a period of time. However, not all of them work indefinitely. Many breast implants develop hard lumps which may be the result of scarring. Sometimes the silicone gel leaks and causes lumps or migrates to lymph nodes under the armpit, forming a hard lump. Scarring, infection, and severe inflammatory reactions can develop and some implants have to be removed. Occasionally, a contracture, or tightening of the tissue around the implant develops and the new mound is not symmetrical with the other breast. This usually has to be surgically repaired.

There is a growing recognition that implants are not quite as inert as once thought, but fortunately, the complications that develop are rare. Still, they can be frightening. An example with a happy ending follows.

I recently saw a woman who developed a lump right next to her silicone prosthesis and she was extremely apprehensive about possible recurrent cancer. A mammogram was done and the radiologist, who examined her, felt the lump was silicone that had leaked from her prosthesis. This was confirmed when the implant was removed and a new one inserted.

Advice for Women Considering Breast Reconstruction Following Mastectomy:

1. Don't be afraid to ask questions. Have the plastic surgeon explain the different types of operations and implants. Discuss the advantages and disadvantages of each.
2. Ask the surgeon if he or she is a board-certified plastic surgeon.
3. Ask the surgeon how many breast reconstructions he or she has done during the past year.
4. Ask the plastic surgeon if you can talk to women who have had breast reconstruction following mastectomy. But remember, results are not the same for all women with different breast cancers and different treatments.
5. Ask to see pictures. Some surgeons do not give out names of patients, but you should be able to look at "before-and-after" photographs of women who have had reconstruction. Look at more than one picture. In particular, you should look at some of the scars that are present after the reconstruction.

SUMMARY

If you want to have breast reconstruction, the time to speak up is *before* the mastectomy. Tell the surgeon who is going to do your mastectomy that you want him to think about the fact that you will be having a reconstruction in the future. In the past, many women got less-than-receptive reactions from their surgeons when they broached this topic and they became discouraged. This has completely changed, as surgical techniques have improved. A woman can feel "complete" again. Women with an implant or muscle-skin graft should know, however, that not all implants are successful. Follow-up examinations are necessary.

QUESTIONS

Q. *What is your criteria for selecting patients for reconstruction?*

A. Each case has to be assessed individually. Reconstruction should not be offered to all mastectomy patients and not all mastectomy patients are interested in having it done. But one criterion is this: the patient should be completely free of metastatic disease. The bones, lungs, liver, and soft tissues should not be involved.

Q. *How is this determined prior to reconstruction?*

A. Chest x-rays, bone, liver, and CT scans, magnetic resonance imaging, and blood tests can be done to determine involvement.

Q. *Do you advise that a delayed or immediate reconstruction be done?*

A. I prefer, if the patient is emotionally stable, she wait a year or more for reconstruction so the mastectomy site will heal properly. This allows the blood supply to grow into the skin flap and for shoulder motion to return to normal. The woman also is less apt to get an infection, which requires removal of the silicone implant.

Q. *What if a sexually active woman who is emotionally disturbed by the absence of her breast wants an immediate reconstruction?*

A. It would depend on the type of tumor she had treated. If she had a large, aggressive tumor I would try to talk her out of it. If the tumor was small and low-grade, then I would allow immediate reconstruction, as it can be a less stressful, rewarding experience for the patient. It should be done in a center where the procedure is done often.

Q. *Are there any other reasons why you prefer to delay reconstruction?*

A. Yes. A silicone implant or muscle transfer can make it more difficult for the doctor to detect recurrent cancer in the chest wall. Most local recurrences occur within 12 to 18 months following surgery, so by waiting a year, doctor and patient can feel more certain they have a "green light" for surgical reconstruction.

Q. *How does a silicone implant interfere with making an early diagnosis of breast cancer or recurrent breast cancer?*

A. Mammography is still the best way to detect cancer or recurrent cancer. The silicone implant causes a radiopaque shadow that interferes with mammographic detail and its ability to evidence small cancers. This suggests that young women who want their breasts made larger (augmentation mammoplasty) should think twice about it if they are in a high-risk group.

Q. Since you can't compress the breast containing a silicone implant to do a mammogram, how does one detect recurrence?

A. Special mammographic techniques are used. Knowledge of the changes after cosmetic surgery is also necessary. Ultrasound can also sometimes be helpful.

Q. Is there any research that suggests that silicone implants delay diagnosis?

A. Yes. Dr. Melvin Silverstein of the Breast Center and Valley Hospital Medical Center in Van Nuys, California, did a study on 753 patients with breast cancer (over a 66-month period). Twenty patients who developed cancer had silicone gel prostheses, and none of these cancers were detected by mammography. The patients eventually presented with a more advanced disease, resulting in a poorer prognosis.[173] Moreover, if you study the patients who develop breast cancer following augmentation mammoplasty and compare them with the nonaugmented group who develop breast cancer, those who have the implants get more advanced and more invasive cancers.

Q. What is a tissue expander implant, and is it better than a routine silicone implant?

A. A regular silicone implant has a fixed size. A tissue expander implant can be injected with saline or other substances to obtain the desired breast size. One recent advancement in implants is the permanent expander implant.

Q. When a silicone implant is used to create a new breast mound, do all patients have a reconstructed nipple?

A. No. Many patients are happy with just the new breast mound, which enables them to have freedom of movement without fear of dislodging the prosthesis. They can wear bathing suits and form-fitting clothing again. Many do not request the additional reconstruction of the nipple. Others want it.

Q. Can complications occur after immediate reconstruction?

A. Yes. Sometimes a wound infection or slough of tissue develops, causing the loss of the skin covering the breast. A major complication can be overwhelming, since postoperative bleeding can also develop. These are reasons why I prefer the patient adjust to the loss of the breast and have delayed reconstruction if they have a reasonable life expectancy and no indication of metastases or recurrence.

Q. Are there any other considerations concerning immediate reconstruction?

A. Today, some women are given adjuvant chemotherapy and/or radiation therapy as part of their treatment regimen. These treatments should be completed prior to reconstruction.

Q. Which women with breast cancer do you advise not to have reconstruction?

A. Those patients in which numerous lymph glands are found to be involved with metastatic cancer. Patients with diffuse metastatic breast cancer to the bones, brain, and lungs are also discouraged from having reconstruction. Women with other serious medical problems are also advised against it.

Q. How do you select a plastic surgeon for your patients to have reconstruction?

A. I usually give them the names of three plastic surgeons so that they may select their own. I prefer to recommend plastic surgeons who are willing and capable of doing all types of reconstructive procedures and avoid those who limit themselves to one or two procedures. I also prefer those who are doing breast surgery frequently; experience counts when you want good cosmetic results.

Q. What are the advantages and disadvantages of the various reconstructive methods after mastectomy?

A. All my breast cancer patients were asked how they felt about the breast reconstruction they had done. I also asked them whether they would have the procedure done again. The patients who were pleased with their reconstruction were the ones that had the simplest procedures, such as the silicone implant. The answer they gave was that they no longer had to worry about the "thing" (external breast prosthesis) being placed in the proper position. They felt their body contour was more normal after the reconstruction.

Q. What did the patients with breast reconstruction object to the most?

A. The main objection to reconstruction came from patients who had musculocutaneous (muscle-skin) island flaps. The latissimus dorsi myocutaneous flap was objected to the most. This is the muscle on the flank and back that is used. Many said they would not have it done again. They did not like the scar on the back, nor the restriction of movement associated with the flap. They objected to the two or three procedures needed for the reconstruction and to the operation (reduction mammoplasty) that often had to be done on the remaining breast. Some patients objected to the cost and others to the multiple scars created by the muscle transposition.

Q. *Should the nipple be removed when doing a mastectomy?*

A. One of the major objections to doing a mastectomy and removing the nipple is that in reconstruction of the breast the woman wants a new nipple constructed. A new nipple is never as good as the original. Here's why. Most breast cancers are infiltrating ductal cancers and the ducts connect with the nipple. If the nipple is left in place the patient is at risk for local recurrence at the site of the retained nipple. This means that rigid criteria have to be used in selecting patients who may qualify for the preservation of the nipple at another site and then using it later in the reconstruction.[188,189]

Q. *Should the reconstructed breast be symmetrical with the remaining breast?*

A. Sometimes this is difficult to achieve because the patient may have a larger remaining breast and a reduction (reduction mammoplasty) has to be done. Since the second breast is at increased risk for cancer, an argument can be made for removing the breast tissue in that breast, followed by a silicone implant.

Q. *Are there any complications to breast reconstruction after mastectomy?*

A. Yes, but as more of these procedures are done, experience is gained and fewer complications occur. In the cases I have seen, most of the complications have occurred in the irradiated cases and in those patients who have had a radical mastectomy with removal of the muscles prior to reconstruction. In the zeal to attempt to eradicate the cancer by surgical means, little soft tissue and thin skin remains for an adequate reconstruction. Postoperative irradiation (prior to reconstruction) reduces the normal circulation to the area and one is more apt to get a slough of the skin flap. Patients with hematological disorders or blood clotting deficiencies are also more likely to get a hematoma (collection of blood) which may lead to an infection and loss of the implant.

Q. *Can radiation therapy be given after a silicone implant?*

A. Yes, and I find that radiation therapy is being used more and more as an adjunctive method of treatment with surgery, particularly when a minimal cancer is found. Chemotherapy is being used more often for patients who do not have cancer-positive lymph glands. This is still slightly controversial and should be discussed with your cancer specialist.

Q. Some doctors have recommended removal of breast tissue (subcutaneous mastectomy) to prevent cancer. Others have advocated mastectomy as a preventive measure in specific types of precancerous lesions. How do you feel about that?

A. Attempting to remove all breast tissue to prevent cancer of the breast has been discussed and written about for many years.[190] The basic problem that has to be faced, however, is whether 100 percent of the breast tissue can be removed when doing a prophylactic subcutaneous mastectomy because if tissue is left behind, then that tissue is at risk to get cancer and may even be at an increased risk.

Q. Can you elaborate further?

A. It is impossible to remove all breast tissue. Breast tissue is always left behind under the nipple and in the tail of spence (axillary tail). Small pieces of breast tissue are also scattered under the skin flaps. The breast is a secreting organ (lactation, milk) and if tissue is left behind it is still going to be affected by hormones (estrogen, progesterone) and can cause problems.

Q. Should a woman discuss costs before having reconstructive procedures done on her breast?

A. Yes. I tell the patient to discuss costs with the plastic surgeon and to ask about various options of treatment and the number of procedures required to accomplish the desired results. In some states the cost of reconstruction after mastectomy is covered by health insurance, but not in all. The cost of reconstruction can be quite expensive in some areas of the country.

Q. How much does breast reconstruction cost?

A. Between $3,000 and $15,000, depending on the number of procedures that have to be done and the center where it is done. You should check with your physician and your insurance company about whether your surgery qualifies for insurance coverage before you have your reconstruction done.

Q. Where can one get advice and counseling before breast reconstruction?

A. The Reach to Recovery Program of the American Cancer Society can provide information to women interested in breast reconstruction. Volunteers who have had reconstruction are available to visit women who are contemplating this type of surgery. No products are endorsed and there is no charge for the service. Some breast surgeons have their own mastectomy patients who work with the physician in counseling women who request reconstruction.

Q. *Which patients are most unhappy with reconstruction?*

A. Those who have a poor self-image to begin with, and expect the surgery to change their life. They may also have emotional problems unrelated to the physical disease that can only be resolved through counseling or psychotherapy.

Q. *What is the latest in breast reconstruction after mastectomy?*

A. Free-flap surgery is a new technique now being used in some academic centers.

Q. *What is free flap surgery?*

A. Free-flap surgery is the use of wedges of fat taken from a mastectomy patient's abdomen, buttocks, or thighs and transferred to the mastectomy site—very small arteries and veins are sewn together to furnish cell nourishment to the breast substitution.

Q. *Who's doing it and how many have been done?*

A. In 1988, approximately 1,300 mastectomy patients had free flap reconstruction done. Persons interested in free flap surgery can call the American Society of Plastic Surgery at 1-800-635-0635.

Q. *Should all mastectomy patients have free flap reconstructions?*

A. No. The procedure is time consuming and technically demanding and is much more expensive.

Q. *Recently some silicone breast implants have been tied to cancer by the Federal Drug Administration.*

A. That is a worrisome problem. The danger may be related to the polyurethane coating placed over some silicone implants that slowly dissolves in the body. I'm sure that a suitable substitute will be developed.

20

Does Your Personality Make You Cancer Prone?

Which comes first, the chicken or the egg? Do you have a personality that makes you more susceptible to cancer and then get it, or do you get cancer and then develop the personality change? There's no definitive evidence that your personality predisposes you to develop cancer, although there is positive evidence that exogenous forces around us may play a big part in whether we get cancer.

This book has discussed many of these outside forces. The *water you drink*, which may contain hazardous waste that produces leukemia; the *food you eat*, which may contain excessive animal fats or harmful preservatives that can cause colon and possibly breast cancer; and *the air you breathe*, which may fill your lungs with pollution, or smoke, that causes lung cancer.

There are other, subtle forces that have a strong effect on the development of one's personality. Parents, teachers, and peers influence you as you grow, and as you become older your personality becomes more fixed. Your ability to adapt to and deal with stress may have something to do with that upbringing. Coincidentally or not, cancer occurs most often in the older age group (the fifth and sixth decades of life), when it is more difficult to change one's personality.

158

In today's society, everyone lives with some degree of stress and one's response and adaptability determines their quality of life and how they will survive.

We know, for instance, that individuals in high-stress jobs are more prone to stomach ulcers, bowel changes (such as diarrhea or constipation), and even heart attacks. Police, who often develop hypertension, are prime examples of those who suffer stress-related maladies. In some states police are afflicted with job-related stress to a point where they are forced to retire early.

People who are nervous, hot-headed, and explosive when challenged have been classified as Type A personalities and are at much greater risk for heart attacks. How a woman responds to the stresses of daily life is part of her personality. If she turns inward without responding directly and constructively to an acute stress, then chronic stress can affect the body system, which is so important to defending against invaders. Emotions, such as the ability to cry, are extremely important in adapting to adversity. Emotions can be volatile and life-threatening at times.

It would be helpful if we were capable of developing a split personality; one to handle stress, and another to deal with everyday, nonstressful situations. However, this doesn't happen. In some cases you have to lash out at others; other cases call for calm and equanimity.

One physiological manifestation of internalizing stress is irritable bowel syndrome, which is seen frequently in women. It is influenced by psychosocial factors and causes diarrhea and/or constipation. The spastic colon seems to occur most often in the overanxious individual, and these people typically seem to be preoccupied with what is happening in the outside world.

There are some suggested disease patterns that predispose an individual to cancer. Ulcerative colitis often progresses to cancer of the colon. Prolonged excessive smoking progresses to cancer of the lung, yet not all heavy smokers get lung cancer. Is there a certain type of personality that is more prone to that type of cancer? When you talk to smokers and try to convince them to stop, their reply is that they can't. "I'm dependent on smoking. I release my tension this way. It keeps my weight down. If I stop smoking I eat too much and become fat." There is no doubt that, in some cases, smoking is associated with a dependent personality.

Excessive alcohol intake is a known causative factor in esophageal cancer and specific character disorders have been associated with this problem. Recent research suggests there may be an inherited gene that predisposes one to alcoholism.

PERSONALITY AND BREAST CANCER

Many studies have been done on breast cancer patients to try to determine specific personality traits that might be associated with the development of the disease. In my practice I have noted no one specific personality linked to women who develop breast cancer.

During the time that I have been treating breast cancer patients, I have noticed that most of these women immediately become depressed once the diagnosis of cancer is made. This hardly seems worth mentioning, but their anxiety increases and in many cases there is guilt and extreme hostility—Why did it happen to me?

Certainly, part of this depression is related to the fear of a possible mastectomy or death. The stress associated with the diagnosis of breast cancer is as acute as it is evident. But is it possible that stress itself preceded the development of the cancer and made the woman more vulnerable to the disease?

In a questionnaire sent to my patients, more than 40 percent with operable breast cancer stated they had either an acute stress (six months) or chronic stress (five years) prior to getting breast cancer. An example of acute stress is the loss of a loved one (death in the family). A chronic stress would be living with an unemployed alcoholic for a long period of time.

The normal physiological mechanisms that are disturbed by psychological input (such as acute or chronic stress), take a big toll on our bodies, and the functions of the immune and hormonal systems are being investigated in relation to stress. Blood changes have been documented with effects on the T cells and B cells. The immune system can become depressed and thus make the individual more susceptible to any type of cancer.

Personal appearance and diet are interrelated with physiological functions, too. Over 50 percent of my patients stated that they were overweight or obese prior to the diagnosis of breast cancer. Hence one can ask the question: Were they under severe stress that caused them to eat excessively to try to compensate? What effect did the obesity have on their personalities? Did they become more withdrawn and reclusive?

Post–Mastectomy Personality Change

A woman's attitude toward her treatment (such as mastectomy) for breast cancer plays a role in how long she will survive. There is a difference in attitudes of the short- and long-term survivor. The psychosocial aspects following mastectomy, indeed, are quite complicated.

The way a woman coped with stress earlier in her life is usually a way of predicting how she will cope with a suspicious breast lump later in life. The psychological response to breast cancer varies tremendously, because the loss of the breast is just the beginning of a patient's stress. Once the mastectomy is done, the woman undergoes a period of rehabilitation and readjustment. Many will not accept the fact that the breast is gone and refuse to look at the place on the body where it once was.

Disbelief and shock sometimes accompany the depression that follows. If immediate reconstruction isn't done, she may be told that reconstruction can be done at a future time to help restore her body image. At this stage, support by the doctor and family members is important. Hospital breast rehabilitation groups and Reach to Recovery volunteer groups who share their experiences with others are sometimes helpful.

Occasionally, radiation therapy or chemotherapy has to be given if the lymph glands are involved, and the patient's anxiety usually increases when told she needs further treatment. Reassurance that these added methods will help surmount the problem are vital.

The problems associated with stress after mastectomy have been relieved somewhat with the increasing early diagnosis of small minimal cancers now being treated by lumpectomy, axillary dissection, and radiation. There is still stress, however. When a woman looks at her breast after lumpectomy she may ask her doctor, "Did you get it all out?" or "Did the radiation kill all the cancer cells? Is radiation going to give me cancer?" These patients frequently need reassurance about this new treatment for breast cancer.

Sometimes the controversies that develop between surgeons, radiation therapists, and medical oncologists about what the best treatment is for each case can lead to added anxiety and increased insecurity for the patient. For example, the recent controversy over whether all breast patients should receive chemotherapy even if their glands are negative, cannot be taken lightly by the cancer specialist. This treatment means six months of expensive chemotherapy drugs plus office visits, which may or may not be covered by the patient's insurance policy. The side effects of nausea and hair loss are added insults to the woman's body image and her attractiveness.

Most breast cancer patients have follow-up visits at regular intervals, usually every three or four months. Patients often express feelings of anxiety when they come for the visit because they're afraid that a recurrence may be found. And, if and when a recurrence is found, what's next on the agenda for treatment? If radiotherapy has already been given, that option is no longer available. If chemotherapy has been given unsuccessfully, some other agent may be tried. If a recurrence develops after limited surgery, a mastectomy may have to be performed, which may be more difficult after radiation treatment.

Recently, I had a patient develop recurrence 14 years after a mastectomy. Her glands were positive at the time of her initial surgery. "Well, doctor," she said, "I've had a good 14 years. I'm sure there are some new treatments that will help keep me alive with a good quality of life."

I replied, "I'm sure there are too!" What I should have told her was that the best treatment was within her—her spirit and attitude were indomitable.

I'll ask the question again. Which came first, the chicken or the egg? Is there a certain type of personality that predisposes one to get cancer, or does the cancer come first and the personality change follow? I believe that question is a two-way street in the etiology and understanding of breast cancer.

21

Stress and the Body's Immune System

The general ability to fight off disease and infection is governed by the body's immune system. Stress is a proven immunity reducer. In research studies so far, stress has been shown to dramatically lessen the body's disease-fighting powers. If you're one of those people who seldom gets a cold, rarely has the flu and has never had a serious illness, chances are that your body has built up a strong defense system against invading bacteria, viruses, and other toxins. More than likely, you pay attention to what you eat and include plenty of immunity-enhancing foods in your diet. You avoid alcohol and caffeine. You avoid anxiety, tension, and other stressful emotions that are known to drain the immune system. You exercise regularly to keep your body organs in tip-top shape and you don't smoke.

As your body ages, its ability to react to stress decreases and advancing age brings with it a decline in immune competence. The incidence of tumors increases. Cancer is more common in elderly people, as are severe infections such as influenza and pneumonia.

The way your body reacts to stress can vary. Acute stress is known to cause heart attacks and strokes in both young and old people. Constant stress can result in peptic ulcers, inflammation of the colon or large bowel (colitis), and changes in the balance of hormones in the body. These reactions are only now becoming understood by physicians and researchers.

Any factor that threatens the health of the body or has an adverse effect on its function can be considered either stress, disease, or worry. This concept was first formulated some 50 years ago by Dr. Hans Selye[191] who clarified for countless other scientists the complex relationships between the brain and various endocrine glands and the manner in which they normally function to protect us from both mental and physical stress. The immune system sometimes fails when stress becomes too intense or too prolonged. Numerous studies have been done linking stress to the body's immune system and, specifically, its cancer-fighting mechanisms.[192,193,194]

THE BODY'S IMMUNE SYSTEM

The body's immune defenses begin with a "stem cell" in the bone marrow, which produces white blood cells. These white blood cells, called leukocytes, "police" the body in a variety of ways. Some migrate to the thymus gland—a large gland near the heart—where they are programmed by the brain to perform different roles. After leaving the thymus, they are called T-lymphocytes and work in two ways: The *helper* cells warn of any intruders or abnormal cells, and the *killer* cells attack the intruder or malignant tissue. Once the intruder is destroyed, the T-lymphocytes stop the process.

Other lymphocytes are programmed outside the thymus and are called B-lymphocytes. They eventually mature into plasma cells, and produce antibodies—chemicals that attack intruding bacteria and viruses. Cancer is believed to invade or somehow alter these defense mechanisms so that uncontrolled division of the abnormal cells occurs and the surrounding tissue is invaded and destroyed. Each individual primary tumor has its own pattern of local behavior and spread; for example, bone metastases are very common in breast cancer but very rare in cancer of the ovary.

The role of stress and its relationship to the immune system is a complicated one.[195,196,197] An extensive network of bodily responses is involved, in which specific areas of the brain, in conjunction with the endocrine glands, affect the biological mechanisms that are necessary for the body to ward off invasion. During acute and chronic stress, the adrenal gland releases cortisone, which can depress the immune defenses of the body. The degree to which this occurs depends upon the individual and how that individual copes with the stress.

Other factors affect the immune system as well.[198] Obesity and improper diet greatly lower the cancer-fighting mechanisms,[199,200,201] particularly in breast cancer. In studies of women with breast cancer, a high number were immune-deficient. Why they were is difficult to determine. One factor that creates an immune-deficient state is hormones. Radiotherapy[202] and chemotherapy also are known to reduce the T-lymphocytes and suppress the immune system. Prolonged immunosuppressive drugs that are used in organ transplants can suppress the immune system so that a cancer can develop.[203,204] Patients with AIDS syndrome eventually become totally immune-deficient and often die from Kaposi's sarcoma (a cancer).

Since stress plays a role in the aging process and diet may affect one's response to aging, the effect of food restriction on aging has been the subject of intensive investigations. Low caloric intake has an effect on life expectancy. A number of animal studies have shown that animals with restricted caloric intake have much longer life spans than those that are allowed to eat at will. The prolonged life span in diet-restricted animals is related to preservation of the immune function, and the incidence of tumors is greatly reduced in those animals.

Vegetarians are known to have fewer malignant tumors, such as breast and colon cancer, and also live longer. Others, who eat high levels of animal fat with increased triglycerides, have an increased incidence of breast and colon cancer.

But not all stress is bad. There are circumstances under which it alerts the body's defenses so it can better protect itself against infection, cancer, and other diseases.

There is a small gland at the base of the brain (pituitary) which plays a key role in the stress syndrome. This master gland secretes chemicals (hormones) into the bloodstream, which in turn affect other glands in the body (adrenal and thyroid glands). The adrenal gland releases cortisone and catecholamines (adrenalin-like substances). These hormones have a pronounced effect on specific organs and tissues. The pituitary-adrenal axis is one of the main reactors when stress from stimulus, such as cancer, threatens the human body.

In chronic psychogenic stress, the pituitary-adrenal axis is stimulated excessively and the release of adrenalin-like substances and cortisone has a marked immunosuppressive effect. The blood-response B- and T-lymphocytes that are necessary for healthy immune responses are reduced by chronic psychogenic stress, making a woman more susceptible and vulnerable to breast cancer.

The pituitary gland also secretes two other chemicals that are necessary for a healthy immune system—the growth hormone (GH) and the thyroid stimulating hormone (TSH). TSH acts to produce hormones of the thyroid, which is one of the glands necessary to maintain normal healthy metabolic function in the human body. Thyroid disease, particularly hyperthyroidism, is more common in the female and when this occurs the gland frequently hypertrophies (gets bigger). The enlarged gland can easily be seen in the neck. This is believed by some to be a stress response in the gland.

Depressive illness, too, tends to be associated with reduced immune response. Depressed patients produce less thyroid-stimulating hormone (TSH) than nondepressed patients and the thyroid does not function properly.

WOMEN AND STRESS

Why are some women more immune than others to breast cancer? Why are they better able to cope with stress? The answer to these related questions can be revealing. Heredity plays a part, as does environment and lifestyle. Some women simply can't relax. They know they should, but when they try, the results are unproductive. Although few of us really know how to relax or how to benefit from relaxation, the benefits may be considerable indeed, because relaxation can help prevent headaches, hypertension, ulcers, and even cancer.

Diet and exercise are important, too. By making wise eating choices, you may be able to fortify your natural defenses and prevent many of the problems that are caused by an immune system breakdown. Studies show exercise is at least as effective as any pill in coping with stress. Women still outnumber men about two to one in taking tranquilizers, but exercise may be changing how we deal with chronic emotional problems.

Several new studies indicate that during extended exercise, a chemical substance called endorphins is released in the brain, which acts as a natural tranquilizer. Strenuous exercise—running, bike riding, jumping rope—relaxes your muscles and makes you less anxious and uptight. Even walking helps. Exercise regularly, at least three times a week, and you may begin to feel more relaxed and able to make positive changes in your life, without any harmful side effects. It will also help build up your body to its maximum immunity capability.

Among patients with possible breast cancer, stress has a pronounced effect on both immunity and recovery. Women worry about whether a lump is benign or cancerous, what kind of surgery they will need, and how it will affect their sexual relationship. The tremendous number of unknowns exacerbates any pre-existing feelings of anxiety. Among my patients with breast cancer the survival rate was highest (75 percent) among those who exhibited a spirit of willingness and desire to fight the disease and survive. Those patients who felt helpless and hopeless from the beginning of their treatment were unable to cope, and their survival time was markedly diminished.

And while stress inhibited their ability to respond to their cancer, it also played a big role in its onset. Nearly half of them said they had undergone some stress prior to the diagnosis of breast cancer. I found the type of stress was significant. Family problems or divorce headed the list of stressful situations, followed by alcoholism, loss of a loved one, physical or mental illness in the family, loss of a job, a move from home, and depression. Some were not able to handle such stress and it contributed to the onset of breast cancer as the following two case histories illustrate:

A woman with no children—but in a purportedly happy marriage— suffers in silence as her husband turns increasingly to alcohol and eventually loses his job. Unable to cope with her chronic stress over his condition, she seeks a divorce and later marries a successful businessman. The business winds up in bankruptcy. She develops cancer of the breast despite having no family history of cancer.

When she is questioned about the lump in her left breast she admits to having noticed it nine months before the mammogram was done, but that her physician told her it was nothing to worry about. A subsequent biopsy revealed an invasive ductal carcinoma with positive hormone receptors. She had a modified mastectomy. This woman has since had breast reconstruction and is alive and well.

In the second case, a young woman with two children suffers through an unhappy marriage, thyroid problems (requiring two operations), a nasty divorce, and her mother's death from a stroke at age 61. Following the second operation, she is treated with drugs and told her thyroid gland should be removed. Six years after that operation a lump appears in her left breast and a mammogram reveals a carcinoma. A modified mastectomy with axillary dissection was done and this revealed involvement of the lymph nodes.

There can be no doubt that a lifetime of stress plus the chronic thyroiditis (in itself an abnormal immune response) contributed to the onset of breast cancer in this young woman. It is not yet known why the body loses its ability to distinguish between healthy and malignant tissues, but there is evidence that stress, along with other factors, can be linked directly to the destruction of tissues by the body's own antibodies.

TAMING RUNAWAY STRESS

It is impossible to measure the negative influence of stress in our society on our bodies, but many physicians, including myself, believe that stress, through biological mechanisms, enhances the risk of serious illness ranging from heart attack to cancer. Not everyone can afford long-term psychotherapy to help alleviate stress or anxiety. However, here are some proven methods of nonmedical intervention you can use to tame runaway stress and its consequences:

Meditation is a proven stress reducer. In every study so far, it has dramatically reduced anxiety in the majority of subjects tested. Begin by meditating five minutes a day, and increase gradually until you can comfortably meditate for 20 minutes. While meditating, your mind will remain alert, but your heart and respiration rate will drop to what it would be after seven hours of sleep. When you complete your daily meditation, you'll feel more alert, refreshed, and able to cope.

Anger, which differs from stress, can help fight cancer too. In my study of patients with breast cancer, those women who were visibly angry about having cancer—they openly resented the disease—seemed to survive longer than patients who tried to cope with their cancer by showing a false, brave face to the world. By releasing their anger, cancer patients may provoke changes in their body chemistry that help fight the disease.

Wackiness. When periods of stress and symptoms of tension arise, some psychologists believe that it is healthier to stop worrying and to take a completely different tack. We've all got a bit of outrageousness lurking beneath our sometimes overly controlled exteriors, and it can be healthy and tension-relieving to let a little of it surface. Anything will do as long as it's fun, but harmless (to yourself and others). Breaking out of your normal routine through a little wackiness isn't difficult. Most important, laughter can help you take the world and yourself less seriously and, by doing so, ease some of those stressful feelings.

Hobbies.   Brains, like bodies, need exercise if they are to function properly and control stress. Don't be afraid to try something new, completely off your beaten path, like needlepoint, painting, sculpting, or any of a number of hobbies you may have always wanted to try. Start an indoor garden. Buy an aquarium. Do anything—but do it regularly. Many women feel guilty when they're not doing something productive, but the experts reassure us that recreation is neither inactive nor self-indulgent. It may well be an important key to safeguarding your mental and physical health.

Tranquilizers.   During the past several years, there has been a growing concern about the indiscriminate use of tranquilizers. While these drugs do not necessarily have a place in the treatment of all patients experiencing stress, or who have anxiety in their lives, it is likewise important to recognize that stress is a major health hazard and no woman should feel guilty or inferior for taking tranquilizers in prescribed doses. Open and trusting communication between you and your doctor regarding the use of these medications, their limitations, and their hazards is essential.

SUMMARY

It is now clear that reciprocal connections between the brain and the immune system play an important role in the body's coordinated response to infection and tumor genesis. Whatever uses will be found for interferon and other stimulants of the body's immune system will doubtless arise out of a growing number of studies in endocrinology and immunology. Theories, some wildly imaginative, still outnumber facts in many areas. Only when a way has been found to destroy the last cancer cell in the last victim can it truly be said that the science of cancer care is complete.

An understanding of the immune system and how it functions to destroy invaders will eventually give us that answer. Until that time you can start making adjustments in your diet, exercise, and everyday living habits that will build up your body and mind to maximum immunity capabilities.

QUESTIONS

Q. *Are there any easy ways to combat stress?*

A. Definitely. Despite all that has been written about the subject, the role of stress and disease is becoming better understood. The bottom line on stress management is to do what makes you feel better. Try taking a hot bath or a 15-minute walk. It can do more good for an unhappy but otherwise healthy person than all the medicine and psychology in the world.

Q. *How can you avoid stress?*

A. Not all stress can be avoided; it's an inescapable part of everyday life. However, acute or chronic stress is something to be aware of. Ask yourself if your expression is always serious, or if you have a frown on your face even when relaxing. Do you often clench your fists or jaw, or frequently seem worried or preoccupied with one problem or another? Why not express the feelings you have openly and learn to accept them?

Q. *Is there a simple explanation for the role of the immune system in stress?*

A. Not really. It's quite complicated. The brain (autonomic nervous system), endocrine system (glands, hormones) and immune system, (secretory products) with such components as the lymphokines, interleukins and interferons all have special coordinated roles in response to stress. The immune system receives regulatory signals from the brain in response to stress and feeds back its own programmed responses.

Q. *What if the stress is too strong or too prolonged?*

A. Then the immune system wears out and the host (body) becomes more susceptible to disease. The body's response to the AIDS virus, which frequently causes cancer, is a good example.

Q. *Does heredity play a role in immunity?*

A. Yes, to a degree. Some inherited diseases such as colon polyps and hypogammaglobulinemia are known to impair the body's immune system. There are also acquired defects when there is no family-related predisposition toward immune-system dysfunction, and there is a higher risk of cancer in these patients.

Q. *Is inflammatory bowel disease related to stress?*

A. Stress may not be the initiating factor, but is believed to play a role. Psychosomatic factors can influence the course of the disease, too. The link between stress and the inflammatory process may be through the neuroendocrine-immune axis.

Q. *Is ulcerative colitis related to stress, or to cancer?*

A. That's difficult to say. Genetic, psychosomatic and immunologic theories have been postulated. Cancer of the colon affects patients with ulcerative colitis at a rate 30 times greater than the general population.

Q. *What is meant by "active" and "passive" immunity?*

A. When a woman's body has generated the substances that will protect her from disease she is said to have active immunity. When we speak of passive immunity, we refer to the immunity developed through injection of antibodies which have been created in the body of another person or the laboratory. Passive immunity usually doesn't last very long.

Q. *Can immunotherapy be used to treat breast cancer?*

A. Certainly. No other branch of oncology or cancer treatment has expanded more rapidly or produced more profound effects on the control of this disease. Our knowledge about the agents used to stimulate the immune system has had the side effect of revealing to scientists and clinicians vast new unexplored areas of immunotherapy.

Q. *Are there many such immunostimulant drugs?*

A. Yes, but not all display sufficient antitumor capabilities to justify prescribing them routinely. The broader hope, obviously, is that some as-yet-undiscovered chemical agents, synthetic hormones, or immune-enhancing agents may prove capable of producing much longer or even permanent remissions, not only of breast cancers but other forms of cancer as well.

22

Cancer and the Foods You Eat

In today's society, most families have two wage earners because of the complexities and economics necessary to survive. This means that many women have a full- or part-time job to help pay living costs and children's college tuitions.

Arriving at home, after a busy day at the office, the television is often turned on or newspapers read. In either medium, everyone is bombarded with advertisements related to ways to keep healthy: avoid stress, get plenty of exercise, and eat nutritious foods.

You may have had a terrible day at work, complicated by unprecedented levels of stress, and you wonder if mass psychosis is sweeping the area because of the bizarre telephone calls you had to handle. You've had it! You vent your rage at your spouse. You might even reach for a drink or pick up an extra cigarette, but it doesn't help.

Stop. Think it through. Maybe exercise will help, riding a bike or jogging after work, or during lunch. How can you exercise in an office setting? Sitting at a desk pounding a typewriter or looking at a computer screen doesn't pass muster for healthy physical exertion. And having to answer that darn telephone doesn't help either.

172

You feel beset. How can you solve all the problems that come up every day? Your boss doesn't help. He or she has a different set of problems. So what should you do, buy a prayer rug? Consult a psychologist?

Suddenly your attention is turned to the television screen—a famous basketball player is telling you that to stay healthy you should eat Wheaties. Another advertisement playfully lampoons a cereal called Nut 'n Honey. An idea begins to germinate—maybe there is something to foods that help you handle stress, prevent heart disease, and cancer. You hear that oat bran is good for lowering your cholesterol. But an article in a famous medical journal says that oat bran isn't all that great. It does give you more fiber and may help prevent cancer of the colon, but another advertisement shows some Eskimos dining in their igloo in Alaska and states that all that fish oil the Eskimos eat prevents heart attacks. (What the advertisement doesn't tell you is that Eskimos have a high incidence of gallbladder disease.)

We've had our brains pulverized with advertisements extolling the health benefits of certain foods. Where do we start? What do we do? Do we read the labels on the back of health food products? Are all those advertisements telling us the truth?

Well, you can rush down to the corner grocery store, push a cart through the aisles, and load up on health foods. However, you need to be selective in what you buy because of your budget.

You also may have a personal interest in preventing a certain disease through your diet. Your dad may have died of heart disease and your grandmother may have had cancer. Uncle Joe had severe rheumatoid arthritis and Aunt Sarah developed osteoporosis and fractured her spine. What foods should you eat to forestall the onset of these diseases, and, while we're on the topic, what foods play a role in preventing breast cancer?

You've heard the saying, "You are what you eat." You've also been told to eat a well-balanced diet. Who's got time to cook and eat a well-balanced diet? It's obvious that everyone doesn't eat the same food. Women are particularly conscious of the foods they eat and their personal appearance is very important to them. Dieting is part of their daily regimen—more women diet than men.

As a woman approaches menopause, there is a tendency to put on weight and attitudes may change. If she becomes frustrated or unhappy with her lifestyle, she may use eating as a method to relieve that frustration. Don't do it! Excessive consumption of foods like fudge, peanut butter, and particularly animal fat will increase your cholesterol levels and triglycerides so that not only will you be at increased risk for heart attacks, but also breast and colon cancer.

When a woman begins menopause her hormones change, the amount of exercise she gets may decrease, and the middle-age "spread" can become noticeable and alarming. I urge women to reassess what is happening to them and decide to watch their diet, maintain a daily exercise regimen, and try to prevent the onset of weight gain.

Many factors contribute to breast cancer. Diet has been suspected as a major cause.[205] The link between nutrition and breast cancer is very strong. Our tendency to consume fatty foods at a young age (which is increasing) may be extremely hazardous in the future. In countries like Japan, where fatty meat is not the main source of protein, breast cancer rates drop significantly.[206,207,208] By contrast, the daily fat intake in the United States is three to four times greater than Japan's. In Japan, fish and staples other than beef are eaten, thus lowering significantly the risk of getting breast cancer.

Increased dietary fat intake also increases the insulin requirement to maintain sugar metabolic equilibrium and probably causes the body's estrogen level to increase, which places a woman at greater risk for breast cancer.

In contrast, Japanese women have much lower levels of estrogen than American women. When Japanese women, however, move to this country and change their lifestyle, consumption of dietary fat increases and their incidence of breast cancer also increases, approaching the level of American women.[209]

I asked all my breast cancer patients about their dietary habits and weight. Over 50 percent were overweight and admitted to trying to lose weight by unusual dietary methods. The overweight women with breast cancer admitted they liked specific foods; steak, beef, and hamburger were mentioned most often (by more than 45 percent), suggesting that high beef consumption, which often has a high concentration of triglycerides, may be a factor in the development of breast cancer.

The socioeconomic factors associated with breast cancer are obvious. One must be able to afford the cost of a diet rich in fats and cholesterol (beef, milk, protein, etc.)—typical in the U.S. and Europe.

There are numerous theories about why a high-fat diet is unhealthy and why obese women are more inclined to develop cancer of the breast and uterus than lean women. Perhaps such foods promote the secretion of the hormone prolactin in the breast or carry possible carcinogens that feed cancer cells, or modify the body's immune mechanisms so that it cannot defend itself against breast cancer. Perhaps fat itself is cancer-causing. Whatever the reasons, we cannot escape the fact that poor nutrition is a principal risk factor in the development of breast cancer.

Recently, nutritionists suggested that the consumption of certain foods may help prevent cancer. For instance, people who eat cabbage have a lower incidence of cancer than people who don't. Cabbage and other cruciferous vegetables, such as broccoli and brussels sprouts, are considered good sources of fiber and vitamins. It is not known which components in these vegetables help prevent cancer.

It has also been found that foods rich in beta-carotene, which the body converts to vitamin A, are associated with lower risk of cancers of all kinds. Foods high in vitamin A content include apricots, peaches, citrus fruits, and deep yellow vegetables such as carrots, yellow turnips, and winter squash.

Diet, Nutrition and Cancer, published by the National Academy Press in 1982,[210] is an excellent reference for those wanting to study in depth the role of diet and nutrition in cancer. This book can be obtained from U.S. Government Services. A more recent book *Diet and Health*, published by the National Academy Press in 1989,[211] is also recommended.

Before storming the supermarket for cabbage, carrots, or other foods that might prevent cancer, it's important to understand what is meant by good nutrition and how it relates to women and breast cancer. For one thing, not all foods are as good as we think they are, and other supposedly "natural" foods may contain more additives and calories than we would expect.

The important thing is to exercise prudence and common sense about what you eat—try taking in fewer calories and less fat. Each day eat some whole-grain cereals, fruits, and vegetables, particularly those high in vitamin C and beta-carotene. Cut down on your intake of pickled foods and smoked foods like sausages, bacon, and hot dogs. Avoid excessive alcohol, particularly if you smoke cigarettes. This boosts the risk of cancer in women who are not otherwise at risk.

It's a matter of controversy as to whether you should add vitamin supplements to your diet to prevent cancer. While all claims cannot be proved, few will argue that a woman who adds vitamin supplements to a balanced diet low in fats will probably feel and be healthier. She may also be reducing her cancer risk. This was first demonstrated by Dr. Linus Pauling[212] a decade ago in his studies of vitamin C and cancer prevention, and in studies done on other vitamins since then.

Research has shown that specific vitamins, whether in the foods we eat or as tablets, can inhibit the growth of cancer cells and help in the healing of precancerous lesions.[213,214] There is little evidence, however, that massive doses of these same vitamins can be more effective in treating patients with advanced stages of cancer. For example, in my study of breast cancer patients, 46 percent said they took vitamin C or a multivitamin supplement daily. One-third reported they took vitamin E supplements.

CAFFEINE AND FOOD ADDITIVES

It may be difficult to believe, but not everything we eat causes cancer. Caffeine, for example, is usually ingested in beverages and has been linked to fibrocystic disease,[215,216] which some believe is a precursor to cancer. However, there is little evidence to support such findings. Other types of benign breast disease may have a more malignant potential (atypia, hyperplasia, papillomotosis).

The caffeine in coffee, tea, and cola drinks is harmful to people with a heart condition or peptic ulcers because it increases the flow of blood to the heart and increases the amount of acid and pepsin in the stomach. It is also a lipolytic agent which helps to break down fats and in this way can lead to an increase in your weight. Caffeine may also cause birth defects if pregnant women drink it in substantial amounts. Gradually try to limit your intake. Don't go cold turkey—that can disrupt the body's cycle and cause headaches. Instead, get yourself down to one cup a day.

People have become so concerned about the harmful things in food that it might be reassuring to know there are many foods that are good for you. Sweet acidophilus milk, for example, may prevent breast cancer. Tests of this low-fat milk indicate that it helps lower the levels of enzymes responsible for generating carcinogens and may limit circulation of estrogen and cholesterol, both suspected cancer-causing agents. There's more than a grain of truth to high-fiber diet claims, perhaps because chewy fiber foods take longer to eat and create a feeling of fullness, thereby aiding in weight control.

Food additives are another story. These have little or no nutritive value and some are actually suspected carcinogens. Yet only a small proportion of these substances are actually tested to see if they do cause cancer. They are used to make food look more appealing (red dye in beef), taste better (saccharin, caramel), or stay fresh longer. The only way you can be sure foods are "natural" is to buy fresh fruits, vegetables, meats, dairy products, and fish.

Listing ingredients on most foods is mandatory, but the words can be twisted to convey whatever the manufacturer wants. According to the U.S. Department of Agriculture, many foods advertised as "natural" contain additives, preservatives, artificial coloring, or other less-than-wholesome ingredients. The damning evidence against unsaturated fatty acids, such as those in sunflower oil, may be just as incriminating as saturated fats such as butter and lard. Check food labels for all ingredients and suspicious additives as well as the number of calories and vitamin and mineral content.

Studies have shown that as our bodies age we become more susceptible to the harmful effects of food additives, fatty foods, and an improper diet. This is especially true for the woman at menopause who is more at risk of developing breast cancer. Keeping weight down and getting sufficient vitamins are doubly important at this often-stressful time.

STRESS AND ALCOHOL

Stress can play a role in the etiology of breast cancer, just as it is known to in other diseases. And—this is important—certain foods are known to increase or decrease stress in the same way they might cause allergies. Research on diet-related behavior suggests that what we eat can affect our moods by altering certain brain chemicals or neurotransmitters. Even skeptics agree that people who are well-nourished tend to feel better and have more energy. Clearly, if you want better mental health, you can't ignore your diet.

The best diet plan for mental and physical health contains fresh, unprocessed foods. You should limit consumption of animal protein because of its high fat content. Emphasize vegetables, fruits, whole grains, and nuts. These foods are the best sources of mood-stabilizing vitamins and minerals such as magnesium, calcium, and the B-vitamins. They also release sugar slowly and, consequently, help keep one's energy levels and temper even. Fresh saltwater fish is an excellent source of protein without high fat content.

Drinking alcohol can also be harmful if you want to stay on an even keel. Alcohol stimulates the body's production of insulin, affecting blood sugar, energy, and mood, similar to those produced by eating processed foods. A hospital study has shown a definite link between alcohol and breast cancer in patients who were heavy drinkers.[217]

Some of the reasons why alcohol puts women at risk to develop breast cancer are known, while others are only now being investigated.[218] For one thing, alcoholic drinks are high in calories, which can lead to obesity and liver damage. The liver, as we know, is the body's enzyme-producing factory and a vital part of its defense mechanisms against cancer.

Alcoholic drinks also contain nitrosamines, additives, and preservatives that are known or suspected carcinogens. The World Health Organization,[219] in fact, has seen fit to label excessive consumption of alcoholic beverages as a causative factor in many types of cancer. The body is only able to metabolize about one ounce of whiskey per hour. Several drinks in a short time causes a marked increase in blood alcohol concentration with all of the obvious toxic effects.

No one, specific alcoholic beverage is better than another. Beer drinkers are just as likely to develop cancer as those who favor gin or scotch. Mixed drinks are no less toxic than whiskey on the rocks. It's the total alcohol content and not the type of beverage that causes the damage and the best advice is to drink either in moderation or not at all. This is particularly true for pregnant women, since as little as one ounce of alcohol a day can lead to a significant decrease in a baby's birth weight, and increases the likelihood of miscarriage.

If you're interested in finding out what your favorite libation includes (few companies freely disclose what they put in their products) the booklet *Chemical Additives in Booze* can be obtained from the Center for Science in the Public Interest (see Appendix B). This organization has been trying since 1972 to get the federal government to require complete ingredient listings on alcoholic beverages.

DIET AND EXERCISE

You should, of course, exercise regularly to get all the benefits of a proper diet. High blood pressure, cardiac disease, or chronic lung problems may rule out some forms of exercise. Your previous medical history may also limit your athletic schedule, but the odds are that your doctor won't raise any barriers to your exercising.

Research shows that such a program can also enable your body to cope better with stress, and can contribute to a speedier recovery from everyday infections. The body is an efficient factory for disposing of all kinds of harmful chemicals if the organs are functioning properly. Muscles, heart, and lungs all depend on food and exercise to work efficiently and eliminate waste products. Bone marrow and lymph tissue, in particular, play an important role in cancer prevention.

Lymph glands, which are found in many parts of the body, act as a filtering system against infection or disease and are a source of lymphocytes (white blood cells), which produce cancer antibodies. Lymph passes through a series of filters, or nodes, and is ultimately returned to the bloodstream. All that one needs to do to have healthy lymph, blood, and bone marrow is to maintain an adequate diet, avoid toxic substances, and exercise to keep the body healthy and prevent infections. Something else to remember is that while one in nine women develop breast cancer, eight do not. Something is protecting those eight women, and part of that something could be in the foods they eat and their lifestyle.

SUMMARY

Experts tell us that the cause of some cancers may be what we eat. How can you find out what particular foods are the cause and what foods you should eat? The best tactic is to be your own cancer detective. Read food labels for total calories, additives, and other ingredients. Purchase *fresh* vegetables, fruits, fish, and meats whenever you can. Avoid alcohol in excessive quantities so that your body is better able to function as an immune system. Even more important, get sufficient exercise and avoid excessive weight gain.

QUESTIONS

Q. What are some of the foods that may be linked to cancer prevention?
A. The National Cancer Institute has identified quite a few: citrus fruits, garlic, parsley, licorice root extract, are some of them.

Q. How does garlic help prevent cancer?
A. Raw garlic, when dried, extracted, and aged to form a powder, can enter the body's cells to increase the immune response. The immune system is extremely important in fighting cancer.

Q. Does yogurt fight cancer?
A. Yes and no. Yogurt has been shown to fight bacteria. The role that bacteria and viruses play in producing cancer is dramatically portrayed by the megavirus producing AIDS. It completely knocks out the immune system and the patient dies from an overwhelming infection or a cancer known as Kaposi's sarcoma.

Q. *How does licorice prevent cancer?*

A. Many scientists feel that cancer starts out as a cell mutation—a cell that goes haywire and multiplies rapidly. Licorice has been shown to help protect the liver and slow cell mutation.

Q. *Why all the publicity about vitamin E?*

A. Several studies showed that vitamin E helped to relieve the pain associated with fibrocystic breast disease. However, the antioxidant properties of this substance (tocopherol) do not work in all patients and it is already fairly widely distributed in any well-balanced diet.

Q. *Does vitamin E have other effects on the body?*

A. Vitamin E has been called the fertility vitamin and some women have felt that their ovarian function has been stimulated by the use of it.

Q. *What about megadoses of vitamins?*

A. Massive doses of any vitamin or mineral can create a toxic overload. Some of the possible effects are headaches, blurred vision, and impaired hormonal action and blood circulation.[220,221] If a dose is large enough, vitamins stop acting like foods and start acting like drugs.

Q. *Are some vitamins better than others?*

A. It depends. The vitamins to be wary of are A, D, and E. These are not water soluble, and are not excreted in daily urine. Instead, they build up in the body and an overdose can be harmful.

Q. *Recently, vitamin-D deficiency has been linked to three or four of our most frequent cancers—colon and breast cancers among them.[222] How does it work?*

A. The precise mechanism for vitamin D, and sunlight's protective effect is unknown, although there is evidence that it relates to calcium metabolism. Vitamin D also might have more direct anticarcinogenic properties.

Q. *Is there any other evidence?*

A. Yes. In the sunny climates of the Caribbean (Central America) there are very low rates of colon and breast cancer. The incidence is nearly zero in equatorial Africa. Where sun exposure decreases, the incidence abruptly increases.

Q. *What minerals help to prevent breast cancer?*

A. Potassium is one—invisible, tasteless, but vital. When we lower our sodium intake while increasing potassium, blood pressure is reduced because potassium discourages the body from retaining water. Calcium and magnesium also help in blood circulation and bone marrow production. Good sources of all three are bananas, chicken, cantaloupes, skim milk, yogurt, and green leafy vegetables.

Q. *You don't mention beef. Is there a reason?*

A. Yes. Beef is a major source of saturated fats and barbecuing generates small amounts of carcinogens. The evidence from countries where people consume far less beef than we do in the United States is just too dramatic to ignore.

Q. *Is the food in fast food restaurants good for you?*

A. Most of the food in fast food restaurants is fried: hamburgers, french fries, chicken, fish, and so on. These foods contain a lot of fats and calories. There also may be high amounts of sodium and saturated fats used in the cooking process. Moderation should prevail in eating these foods.

Q. *What should we eat instead of beef?*

A. We should be eating more fish, chicken, and fresh vegetables, especially those high in B and C vitamins. A deficiency of vitamin B affects nearly all body tissues, particularly those containing rapidly dividing cells. Vitamin C helps maintain healthy tissue and the integrity of cell walls.

Q. *Why do you seem to play down cholesterol?*

A. It's not the cholesterol content but the total amount of fat in the diet that contributes to breast cancer. This leads to increased free fatty acid levels (triglycerides) which impair the body's immune mechanisms.

Q. *Should one drink only decaffeinated coffee?*

A. Not necessarily. The solvents used to remove caffeine from coffee are often left behind in the coffee and some of them are known or suspected carcinogens. Studies of decaffeinated coffee indicate that it actually *increases* the output of harmful gastric acids.

Q. *Do you think caffeine causes fibrocystic disease or breast cancer?*

A. Not at all. I reviewed all my cases with a proven tissue diagnosis of fibrocystic disease (500 cases) and almost 50 percent drank less than two cups of coffee a day and still got fibrocystic disease. Less than one percent went on to develop breast cancer.

Q. Are some food additives worse than others?

A. Definitely. We commonly ingest more sodium and sugar than we need and the harmful effects of both are well known. In addition, many of the thousand-or-more flavoring agents in foods are suspected cancer-causing substances. These are often complex combinations of ten or more different ingredients.

Q. What should you look for on a food label?

A. The amount of fat or protein, sodium, and carbohydrates. The Food and Drug Administration requires nutrition information panels only on "enriched" or "fortified" foods or on products that make nutritional claims such as "low sodium." However, many manufacturers voluntarily list this information even when their products make no special claims.

Q. What about pesticides and pollutants?

A. Everyone should be concerned about the environment we live in. The water you drink, the food you eat, the air you breathe, are all precious in their natural state and are necessary to maintain a healthy body. Once they become polluted or chemically changed, they become harmful and can cause cancer and other serious problems.

Q. Are the food manufacturers being truthful to the public about the health claims for their food?

A. Not always. The Federal Drug Administration hopes to have specific regulations governing health food claims in the near future.

23

Helping Yourself After Breast Surgery

Depression—the term, let alone the condition, scares a lot of people. Women seem to be affected more than men and some physicians attribute it to the hormonal changes that take place during the monthly menstrual cycle and, in particular, menopause. It's obvious that a woman's mood changes with her period and many women become depressed when menopause approaches. During a woman's lifetime she will experience a short time when, for some reason, she can't cope with a stressful situation and becomes depressed. Others seem to cope outwardly, but inwardly the depression is still present. It has been estimated by the National Institute of Mental Health that as much as 6 percent of the population may be affected with a degree of severe depression during a given year and 60 percent are women—that amounts to over ten million women in this country. Many of these women seek help but the majority don't recognize the symptoms and endure a profound protracted melancholia.

Fortunately, progress is being made with our mental health problems, and they are now openly discussed on television and in newspapers. Patients who have suffered mental illness and depression freely open their souls to the public on talk shows. Magazine articles interview prominent personalities who readily admit to being treated by a therapist, psychologist, or psychiatrist. This openness has provided women with the incentive to seek help.

Breast cancer patients are prime candidates for emotional distress. Women who are told they have a breast lump and need a biopsy (because it may be cancer) usually become depressed. The majority of these patients sleep fitfully until the biopsy is performed. Fortunately, most of them do not have breast cancer. But the acute stress and depression is present until they find this out.

By contrast there is the woman who has been told she *does* have breast cancer. There is immediate shock and depression. Why me? What have I done to deserve this? Will I lose my breast? Will I be half a woman? Will my husband or my partner still love me? What about that new operation that saves the breast? Do I qualify for it? I'm still sexually active. Will I have a partner to share sex with? These are just a few of the questions asked by patients after being told they have breast cancer.

Once the patient has been diagnosed and treated for her breast cancer, she often becomes inquisitive and wants to learn more about her disease. She wants to know how she can help prevent further problems, and if a recurrence does develop, how she can detect it before it becomes life threatening.

The most important development in the treatment of breast cancer during the past 20 years is that the patient seldom has to worry about having a radical mastectomy. Mammography's acceptance in the early 1960's has been a tremendous advance in the detection of breast cancer. Its ability to detect tiny tumors that can't be felt means that the lesion is localized upon discovery and a less radical procedure can often be done to eradicate it. Limited surgery is on the rise.

Patients who have limited surgery are happier because they retain their breast. The breast may be somewhat firmer from the radiation treatment and have scars on it, but the preservation of body contour is obviously appreciated by the woman who qualifies for limited surgery.

There is now more good news about breast cancer treatment. Breast cancer five-year survival rates have increased by approximately 5 percent during the past ten years. The bad news is that the mortality rates for breast cancer have remained the same. This suggests that detection methods (mammography and ultrasound), rather than treatment methods, are improving. Ten years ago, 65 percent of patients who came into my office detected the abnormal lump in their breast themselves. Another 25 percent had the abnormality in their breast detected by their physician (usually an obstetrician or internist). Today, more than 50 percent of breast tumor patients I see in my office have a suspicious, nonpalpable abnormality that was detected by mammography. Many of these patients have needle localization procedures (biopsies) for nonpalpable tumors (less than .5 cm) and a greater number are opting for limited surgery.

Doctors still see large breast cancers and there are still delays in diagnosis. These patients often require modified mastectomies, and while many women regret having the mastectomy after it has been done, they must recognize that it saved their life. The patient should remember, too, that with improved plastic reconstruction methods, the mound of the breast can be replaced with good cosmetic results (see Chapter 19, Breast Reconstruction).

Why is it that some women do better after having a mastectomy than others? The answer is in how they respond to the operation. Some women withdraw from society and become a recluse after a mastectomy. Others continue their daily lives. Still others even seem to thrive on overcoming their infirmity.

A woman's personality, rather than age, determines her ability to recover from the physical and psychological effects of breast surgery. Often doctors are likely to assume—erroneously—that a woman past menopause will not miss one of her breasts. But a woman in her 70's told me that she felt like she'd "lost a good friend" after her mastectomy. Then again, an attractive woman in her early 30's told me if "one boob" was all that kept her marriage together then it would be better to end the marriage.

Defense mechanisms, activated or reactivated by surgery, prove inadequate for some women. They later regret and resent giving their consent for the mastectomy operation. Others report a sense of life "standing still" or being divided into "before" and "after" phases. They are unable to concentrate on the future until the crisis abates and they dare to hope again.

The survivors are those women who remain fully employed and socially active despite surgery, chemotherapy, or radical treatment. For the most part, these women are verbal, confrontational, brave and, at times, scrappy. On occasion they can be hostile, compulsive, and demanding. Rarely are they docile or obsequious. The woman who wants to live and wants to fight will lick the problem. She is unwilling to give up. She will not accept the alternative.

Among the factors agreed upon as personality characteristics of cancer patients who have trouble coping are a tendency to harbor resentment and a marked inability to forgive. Many of these women have a very poor self image and some of them are unable to develop and maintain meaningful long-term relationships. Their grief is usually prolonged and they find it difficult to return to daily activities and resume a normal lifestyle.

Women suffer needlessly as a result of postoperative treatment because their physicians have unknowingly encouraged such negative reactions. When a physician says, in effect, "This may make you sick," many women dutifully follow their doctor's suggestion and proceed to get sick.

It's extremely important for a woman who has a potentially serious breast problem to have confidence in the doctor she has selected to care for her. If a patient comes to me and says she wants a second or third opinion, I encourage her to do so. I tell her to make her own selection so there can be no conflict of opinion. If she decides to have the second or third doctor take care of her, I also encourage this decision. There are so many different opinions today for breast cancer treatment, by outstanding breast cancer specialists. There is usually more than one way to treat a patient. The method of providing 100 percent curability in the treatment of breast cancer has still not been discovered. Therefore, there is room for doubt.

It appears that women who do not like their doctors, or who do not really have faith in the efficacy of the treatment they are getting, tend to become sicker than those who are involved in a working partnership with their physicians. The unhappy patients are also those least likely to follow the physician's directions about follow-up care.

HOW CANCER CAN SPREAD

In order for a breast cancer patient to understand how she should examine her body after surgery or other forms of treatment, it's important to know how cancer spreads. For almost a century, breast cancer was thought to be a single disease that progressed in an orderly fashion from the tumor to the lymph nodes in the armpit and, only then, on to the rest of the body. Early detection has always been thought to be the best hope for surviving the disease.

Recent research, however, shows that breast cancer may be much more complicated. Some scientists now believe that it may well be that breast cancer is a systemic disease from its onset and should be treated as such. Others feel that it starts as a localized disease, a cancer cell that has gone haywire in a localized area and multiplies, growing locally. If treated adequately by surgery, radiation, chemotherapy, or a combination of methods, while confined to the local site, the cancer can be destroyed. Then cancer does not progress on to involve the lymph glands or spread to other organs.

According to an earlier opinion of how tumors spread, a radical mastectomy, which always included removal of the axillary lymph nodes, was the logical treatment. The wider surgical excision and the more tissue removed locally around the breast, including the chest wall muscles, the better chance for a cure. The nodes under the armpit were always removed to prevent further metastases (tumor spread). If the operation failed, it was because it was not radical enough.

Today, the care of the breast cancer patient has evolved into multiple choices because we are detecting breast cancer earlier and if these "minimal cancers" are localized, the breast can be preserved. The problem is that even with our sophisticated methods of detection, we are still unable to determine in all cases if the breast cancer is localized and which patient qualifies for breast conservation surgery.

Mammography and other diagnostic techniques are detecting in situ breast cancer—the earliest, tiniest breast cancer. The treatment of in situ intraductal cancer and in situ lobular cancer of the breast is extremely controversial. There are advocates recommending modified mastectomy, lumpectomy, lumpectomy followed by radiation, lumpectomy without radiation, and so forth—all from sophisticated major cancer centers (See Chapter 12, In Situ Cancer). The arguments for these methods are all good, but because of the major controversies about treatment methods, there is no one best treatment for all cases.

The introduction of limited surgery, such as lumpectomy and axillary dissection followed by radiation therapy, has introduced a new dilemma in follow-up care. It's not easy to monitor these postoperative patients. Some women who have had this type of treatment have expressed doubts about it. "That breast had cancer in it—how can I be sure the radiation got rid of it all?" The breast cancer specialist's job gets tougher here, because the breast becomes more fibrotic (hard) and there's a tendency to do mammograms more often because it's more difficult to palpate a new lump.

I recently saw a patient who had a lumpectomy and axillary dissection followed by radiation. The surgery and radiation were done in another city. The excision margins were adequate and the radiation seemed to be optimal. The patient developed a firm area within a radiation-treated fibrotic breast six months after treatment. A biopsy was done confirming recurrent cancer within the radiated field and a mastectomy was performed. The mastectomy wasn't easy to do because of the fibrosis created by the radiation treatment, which also slowed the healing process.

There's no question that any patient who finds a new lump following any method of treatment should report it to her physician. Chances are that it may be one of several types of lumps or bumps that are quite natural and benign (see Chapter 7, Breast Lumps That Are Not Cancer). However, it is not unusual for the recovering patient to become panicky about the cancer recurring or spreading. She needs to be reassured and, fortunately, today there are a number of tests to do just that. The patient can also be taught what to look for and, even if cancer recurs, it can be successfully treated.

Breast cancer patients are often not told everything they should know about their condition, in the belief that it will cause them anxiety. This may be accurate, but is unfair to the patient, and jeopardizes follow-up treatment, giving women a false sense of security. Some don't like the physician who treated them, and may not seek his advice at all. This makes it important for the patient to choose a professional to see after treatment, one she can talk with freely, whether it's a family doctor, gynecologist, obstetrician, internist, or surgeon.

Learn to trust your doctor and to confide in him. It's important for him to know your feelings as well as your various health complaints. Your doctor should be available at all times to listen.

There are other ways to get help if you need it. The American Cancer Society's Reach to Recovery Program consists of volunteers who have undergone similar breast surgery. Your local Cancer Society is only a phone call away.

WHAT ARE THE SYMPTOMS?

One way to help the patient with breast cancer is to try to help her understand her disease and what to look for to prevent further trouble. Most of my patients want to know more about their disease and what they can do to prevent its recurrence. They are told that tumor spread occurs in three ways: localized invasion of tissue at the site of the operation, through the lymph channels or bloodstream, or across body cavities such as the pleural or peritoneal spaces that line the lung and abdomen. Each individual's primary tumor has its own pattern of spread (metastasis); for example, bone metastasis is very common in breast cancer.

Not all patients can emotionally accept the fact that they may get a local recurrence or that their breast cancer may spread to other areas of their bodies. This type of patient has to be seen more often, and needs reassurance.

Follow-up visits for cancer patients are very important. An appointment is only good if the patient keeps it. It's no good if she cancels and doesn't set up another date.

A woman who has a small cancer of the breast usually does not have to be seen as often in follow-up as one who had a large cancer (larger than 4 cm). If a woman has a large cancer, she is at greater risk for local, regional, or systemic spread. What this means is that the doctor following the patient (the oncologist) should be selective in how he follows the breast cancer patient after surgery, since certain types of breast cancer are more serious than others.

LOCAL RECURRENCES

It's difficult to define what is meant by a local recurrence of a breast cancer. Sometimes it cannot be determined if the doctor is dealing with a local tumor recurrence at the site of the surgery, disease that was left behind and not adequately removed, or spread from another site (metastases).

If a mastectomy has been done there are specific areas that a woman should watch for local tumor recurrence. The site of the surgery should be inspected on a monthly basis by looking in a mirror and gently palpating the surface of the chest wall to feel for any small nodules that may be under the skin surface. If a lump does develop the doctor should be notified. A definitive diagnosis is simple to establish by injecting a local anesthetic and removing the nodule for tissue analysis.

Most of these nodules are benign, and may be small lumps associated with the previous operation (such as silk or other suture material). The lump can be right along the scar and can be a keloid or excessive scar formation.

If a woman has a large, advanced cancer of the breast, one can predict a much higher incidence of local tumor recurrence. The size of the lesion, stage of the disease, and whether the glands are involved at the initial treatment are all important factors in recurrence.

Occasionally it's difficult to detect local recurrence because of special circumstances. For instance, radiation treatments can cause skin to thicken and can mask a secondary tumor. Patients who have had such treatment should be seen more frequently by their physician and have mammograms more often.

The woman who has breast reconstruction surgery should be examined on a regular basis since, because of the implant, it is virtually impossible to examine the chest wall and tissue by breast self-examination. You can't palpate the local area and you can't see it. You also can't compress the breast tissue, as you do for a mammogram to pick up new tumors.

Interpretation of these follow-up mammograms is difficult. Most studies[174] of breast cancer patients agree that if the disease recurs, it will happen within 12 to 18 months after treatment. However, in my experience, tumors have recurred in patients as many as ten or more years after treatment.

Treatment of Local Recurrence

Solitary chest-wall tumor recurrences, if small enough, can be treated by surgical excision if the surgeon can get around the lesion and have clear margins. Surgery, followed by radiation therapy, has to be pursued if clear margins cannot be accomplished. If there are multiple nodules of recurrence, systemic drugs (chemotherapy) may also have to be used.

The local recurrent tissue should always be sent for hormone receptor levels, no matter what the previous receptor levels showed. Receptor levels can change and this can influence treatment.

If the lump turns out to be a local recurrence of the cancer, the patient should be prepared for testing to be sure the lungs, bones, and liver are not involved. In some cases of recurrent cancer, large, local tumors near the sternum that resist radiation therapy have been surgically resected with some success.[223]

REGIONAL RECURRENCE OF BREAST CANCER

Regional tumor recurrence of breast cancer implies that the recurrence develops in the drainage area of the breast and that lymph node spread has occurred. The anatomical distribution of sites for lymph node spread has been previously discussed and, although most of the lymph drainage goes to the axilla (armpit), drainage also goes to the internal mammary lymph node chain beneath the sternum and into the supraclavicular area (above the collarbone).

If a tumor recurrence develops in any of these drainage areas, a lump usually forms and can sometimes be felt. Women are advised to palpate these areas periodically for early detection of recurrence. X-ray imaging techniques are also used, since simple palpation by the patient or doctor is not always accurate. Lymphoscintography (x-ray) can be helpful, particularly in imaging the lymph nodes under the sternum (also known as the internal mammary chain). Other methods used in difficult cases are magnetic resonance imaging and CT scans.

A patient was referred to me from a small hospital because of persistent severe left-arm pain, three years after mastectomy surgery. A surgeon explored an area under the clavicle for a possible recurrence and the tissue diagnosis was fasciitis. A lump and pain persisted. A CT scan revealed a 4 cm lesion at the thoracic outlet, where nerves from the neck area extend beneath the clavicle and out to the arm. The area was re-explored and the tumor (recurrent cancer) was resected. The patient received chemotherapy and postoperative radiation and has been free of pain for five years. In this case, the CT scan was extremely helpful in establishing the diagnosis of recurrent breast cancer.

The important fact for patients to remember is that they should check themselves for recurrence by examining the drainage areas, since early detection usually means salvaging more unaffected tissue. This doesn't mean one has to do it every day—just periodically. Mark it on your calendar if necessary. Patients are advised to check themselves when they are taking a shower, for instance. Many women pick up a suspicious lump before their doctor does.

Evaluation of Lymph Node Spread

If a new lump is found in the drainage area of the breast (axilla or supraclavicular area) a needle aspiration of the lump can be done to examine the tissue. This can be performed by a surgeon or radiologist in the office with local anesthesia, and then the cytopathologist can examine the tissue to determine if a spread of the tumor has occurred.

Occasionally, enlarged glands may develop around the root of the lung and can be seen on x-ray. A radiologist, under x-ray control, will introduce a long biopsy needle to sample the tissue for analysis. This avoids a diagnostic operation and open biopsy.

Treatment of Regional Tumor Recurrence

If a woman develops a regional tumor recurrence, the news isn't always bad but further diagnostic steps should be taken to be certain. Once lymph node spread of breast cancer develops, a complete workup should be done to rule out systemic spread (bone scans, liver scans, CT scans,

MRI, blood tests, etc.) before treating the patient. The usual treatment for regional spread of breast cancer is chemotherapy, radiation therapy, or both. Success with these treatments is quite common.

SYSTEMIC SPREAD OF BREAST CANCER

Systemic spread of breast cancer means that pieces of the primary cancer have broken off and been carried via the lymph channels or bloodstream to other parts of the body. When this happens the news is not good—50 percent of patients will not survive unless treatment is begun immediately. The bones are the most common site of systemic spread, followed by the lungs, liver, and brain. Symptoms are variable and difficult to detect, which is why physicians see these patients frequently. Back pain that persists, aching or painful joints, frequent colds or respiratory ailments, and weight loss are signs of systemic illness that patients are advised to watch for.

Systemic spread of breast cancer is the most serious type, and cure rates are half of those for local or regional metastasis. The survival rate in this group is 15 to 25 percent.

There's reason to believe that these dismal numbers will change in the near future with advances in mammographic and magnetic resonance imaging detection—more and more small, nonpalpable breast cancers are being detected early, as well as metastases to other parts of the body.

Great strides are also being made with chemotherapy and immunotherapy. For example, monoclonal antibodies produced in the body, reproduced in test tubes and then injected into the body, may be able to seek out and destroy cancer cells. Other anticancer drugs such as Interferon and Interleukin also show promise as disease-fighting drugs with the ability to prevent the spread of cancer.

GETTING THE HELP YOU NEED

Not all therapy for the breast cancer patient is medical. Physical therapists can help mastectomy patients with severe swelling or aching muscles to regain the use of their arms. Mild exercises, combined with deep breathing, relaxation, and massage, can strengthen the arm and extend its range of movement in a short time. For women who lack the money or opportunity for private therapy, the YWCA has pioneered a low-cost program called Encore that combines rhythmic exercise, swimming, counseling, and clothing advice for mastectomy patients (see Appendix B).

Other support groups help by sharing the experiences and concerns of women who have had breast cancer. Several of these groups have chapters across the country to help patients and families cope with cancer, improve their quality of life, and combat prejudice against cancer patients. The National Cancer Institute has also funded several projects to study the psychological aspects of breast cancer, including community education, physician education, and crisis counseling. (The psychology of cancer is discussed in more detail in the next chapter, along with how best to cope with the disease.)

Telephone hotlines also exist to help answer questions about breast cancer research, diagnosis, and treatment. One of them, the Cancer Information Service of the National Cancer Institute (800-422-6237), has trained staff members or volunteers who supply accurate and confidential answers to cancer-related questions, and will often mail free publications that are regularly updated. This hotline is also affiliated with the American Cancer Society and regional cancer centers such as Memorial Sloan-Kettering Cancer Center in New York City.

SUMMARY

Until medicine gains a better understanding of the various causes of breast cancer, early detection programs should be acknowledged as providing only limited help. Every woman, and particularly women with breast cancer, need information at one time or another about how breast cancer spreads and treatments to prevent or stop it. The increasing availability of breast-sparing surgery, if they qualify, should encourage women to obtain such information from their family physician, cancer specialist, or support organization. The informed woman usually detects breast cancer early, spares herself pain and trauma, and resumes her life more quickly.

QUESTIONS

Q. *What do you do if a woman is severely depressed after breast cancer surgery?*

A. That varies with each case. First you try to mobilize support, either with the family or outside support groups.

Q. *What if that doesn't seem to work?*

A. The patient can see a psychologist or psychiatrist.

Q. Is there anything new in treating protracted depression after mastectomy?

A. Yes. There is a new miracle drug, Prozac, that seems to help the emotional symptoms of severe depression. Taking the medication along with psychological counseling is quite helpful.

Q. Who should prescribe it?

A. A psychiatrist who knows when and when not to use it.

Q. Is the drug addicting?

A. Not really. Nor does it have the bad side effects that other drugs have.

Q. If a woman has breast cancer should she worry about recurrence?

A. Yes. If she is intelligent and becomes informed about what to look for, she'll be able to pick up a recurrence early.

Q. How can you tell if the cancer has recurred?

A. By the use of mammography and biopsy to determine if a lump is benign or malignant. Other tests such as bone scans, chest x-rays, CT scans, ultrasound, and nuclear magnetic resonance are used as aids in detecting recurrence. Sometimes it's not easy to detect early recurrence.

Q. Should a woman have her ovaries removed to prevent cancer recurrence?

A. Probably not. It was once thought that by removing the ovaries, breast cancer would not recur. This did not prove to be true. However, in those women who had estrogen-dependent tumors with recurrence, surgery for removal of the ovaries or adrenal glands did increase survival time and allowed good palliation. Newer estrogen-blocking drugs have replaced the need for this type of surgery.

Q. Who should take these estrogen-blocking drugs?

A. Such drugs were at first generally prescribed for women who showed evidence of cancer spread. They are increasingly being used as a preventative for recurrence. Tamoxifen is the least toxic oral medication, with few side effects. Estrogen-dependent tumors are easier to treat than those that are not. Tamoxifen has been most effective in postmenopausal women and long-term Tamoxifen definitely delays breast cancer recurrence.

Q. Have there been any recent advances in regard to Tamoxifen?

A. Yes. A team from the University of Wisconsin Cancer Center, which has been studying antiestrogens for more than 20 years, has come up with some new findings.[224] They discovered a line of breast cancer cells that spontaneously change from estrogen-receptor-positive to estrogen-receptor-negative status. This is exactly what happens in patients with recurrent breast cancer. This new discovery will help researchers study breast cancers that have no estrogen receptors (for which there is no conventional therapy).

Q. *What other drugs prevent the spread of cancer?*

A. Cytotoxic agents destroy cancer cells by inhibiting cell division, but dosage must be carefully controlled to protect normal cells, particularly in bone marrow, skin, and fetal tissue. Other drugs being investigated include Interferon, 5-Fluorouracil and Melphalan.

Q. *Are bone marrow transplants being done for breast cancer patients who exhaust their own body's ability to fight the cancer?*

A. This has been considered and tried. Methods to encourage the immune system to reject the tumor are also being tried with limited success. Hospitals are now storing the patient's own bone marrow prior to treatment with some success. Research in this area is ongoing.

Q. *Where can one find out about support groups?*

A. Both the American Cancer Society and National Cancer Institute have offices in a number of cities, and you can call their toll-free hotlincs for additional information (see Appendix B). The YWCA and other local organizations may also offer support and counseling services.

24
Quality of Survival—Coping with Breast Cancer

Matthew 16:26, "For what do it profit a man if he gains the whole world, but suffers the loss of his soul?" What do doctors gain as cancer specialists, if they save a few more patients with breast cancer only to have them lead a life which, for them, is living hell?

In today's society rehabilitation is receiving more emphasis and the evaluation of the quality of survival is being openly discussed. Patients are being asked how they think they are adapting to their treatments. Often, their answers are unpredictable.

The most important human endeavor is the compassion and consideration we have for our fellow man. And in all the mercies of the healing arts, there is no more compelling challenge to demonstrate the deft touch of the surgeon or the sympathetic skill of a physician than giving solace and comfort to those women afflicted with breast cancer.

Lost in the limbo of our earliest cultures is the origin of the relationship between the breast and its symbolic psychosexual significance. However, the sudden discovery of a lump in the breast, with its ensuing anxiety, gives many women the terrifying illusion of irretrievable disenchantment.

196

The breast is undoubtedly a unique feminine symbol, intimately related to beauty, charm and certainly to Hollywood-inspired sex appeal. It also bears the added distinction of being the badge of motherhood.

Let's visualize what a woman might think when she's told she needs a biopsy of a breast lump. Picture in your mind what may be going through her mind. She may have detected the lump herself, possibly in the shower, or her doctor may have found the lump in her breast on routine examination. Her doctor then tells her she needs to see a surgeon. Now she's worried. She wants to see the surgeon immediately. A very tense situation develops. She may have to face several days of waiting for a hospital bed. She's thinking: "Is this cancer or isn't it? What's going to happen to my breast? Am I going to die? What will happen to my family?"

The doctor can provide support for this woman by telling her that most lumps are not cancer. He can reassure her there is now a two-stage method of proceeding with breast cancer treatment. She will need a mammogram first, then a biopsy, and then a skillful pathologist—or team of pathologists—will examine the tissue after it has been removed. If a diagnosis of cancer is established, she will be able to sit down with her doctors, her husband, her family, and friends to discuss her breast care options.

More tiny cancers are being detected by mammography, and more often than not, she will be able to preserve her breast. In those patients who need a mastectomy, they should be informed that reconstruction methods have immensely improved and if everything works out all right, a new breast can be reconstructed.

When the patient is first seen by her breast cancer surgeon, it is his duty to allay her fears, and bolster her morale. He should be completely truthful with his remarks, but the truth should be tempered by moderation. He should not embellish his remarks and go into details about the operative procedure. He should try to direct the patient toward what he believes is the best treatment for her. No two cases are exactly alike and each patient should be treated individually. There also will be conflicts in recommended treatment methods. Second and third opinions are often given. In certain areas of breast cancer treatment, there are gray areas and this should be explained. The breast cancer specialist tries to inform her fully about alternative methods of treatment.

Informed consent means exactly what it says—the patient wishes to be fully informed and comprehensively instructed about her options in treatment in order to select the method she wants. After being as fully informed as possible, she may then consent to or deny the recommended treatment (see chapter 10, Informed Consent).

Major operations are traumatic experiences for patients, and a mastectomy certainly qualifies for that definition. An important sexual organ is being removed. A woman's body is altered. A new image must be rebuilt.

The immediate adaptation to this experience varies. Older women seem to adapt better to the loss of their breast than younger women. It is harder for a young woman to accept the assault that a mastectomy has waged on her body. She is usually sexually active and worries about intimacy with her partner. There are many assumptions about the mastectomy patient, the most common being her feeling that she is "half a woman" and no longer sexually attractive to her partner.

Yes, there is a body contour change when the breast is removed, but how that affects the love relationship may be debated. I asked all my mastectomy patients if their sexual relationship had changed after mastectomy. Twenty percent said it had changed for the worse. But some of these women blamed themselves. They said it was not due to a lack of desire or ardor from their partner, but rather to their own emotional readjustment. They said they became depressed, withdrawn, and unable to continue their daily activities. They lacked self esteem and often refused supportive efforts from family and friends.

Actually, if the man and woman have a strong relationship prior to mastectomy, it is common for that relationship to continue, and many times the male becomes more considerate and affectionate.

I find the quicker the woman faces the reality of the mastectomy, the quicker and easier the adjustment is made. To ignore the situation and treat the woman as though nothing has happened can be psychologically damaging, for she cannot unburden herself of her feelings and this repression may delay her recovery.

Love and communication are the basic ingredients in a good family relationship. When they are present, the shape or absence of breasts becomes unimportant. The brush with death itself often brings couples closer together.

Many husbands and lovers, after their initial shock, respond to their partners nobly. A tall, single, pretty stockbroker I did a mastectomy on when she was 29 years old was depressed following her surgery because she felt she would never have the chance to get married. At the age of 32 she did get married and now has two lovely children. She told me that her sexual relationship is completely normal and happy.

Another woman, 60 years old, told me she missed her breast and was considering reconstruction. "Women live a lot longer than men, you know . . . If my husband dies it will help make me more attractive and appealing." Other patients do not exhibit this kind of buoyant practicality.

This is especially true for unmarried or divorced women, who expect that the loss of a breast will cost them dearly. Perhaps it does, but not as much as one would suppose.

Consider, for example, the following case history of an attractive woman, 41 years old, who said, "My lover took off as soon as my mastectomy was done." She was separated from her husband at the time of the operation and had expressed some doubts about how her new partner would react, since he had told her on more than one occasion that her breasts were beautiful. When asked how she felt now, she said, "It was the best thing that ever happened to me. I found out that he didn't really completely love me. It was strictly a physical relationship. And my new husband is in the waiting room. Would you like to meet him?"

One patient's husband told me, after his wife's mastectomy, that when he looked at his wife, he didn't think of her as missing a breast but missing the cancer that had been in her body. The fact that she had only one breast didn't make him love her any less. He was grateful for the fact that the cancer had been removed, and that their life together could continue.

COPING WITH DEPRESSION

The amount of help a woman gets from her husband, lover, or friends usually depends on the prior quality of their relationship. This is important enough to be a deciding factor in whether she has a short or long depression. Shrouding the operation in secrecy, omitting family members from medical discussions, ignoring a woman's emotions or overprotecting her only impedes help and recovery. Some women vent their anger at the surgeon. Others express disbelief or deny the consequences of the procedure. Outside counseling is often needed in order to overcome these feelings of depression or anxiety.

What are some of the ways a woman can help herself cope after a mastectomy? I find that women who exercise and try to keep their bodies in good shape seem to cope better with the physical and psychological trauma associated with mastectomy. As part of a rest and relaxation treatment (particularly if you're the aggressive, self-driven type), try deep-breathing exercises, walking, or biking. They're good for both your health and your morale and will speed up recovery.

Regular, self-induced relaxation can also be helpful in beating the blues. One way is to try meditation or visualization. These are not new ideas, but what is new is that many physicians, after focusing on the body alone for so long, are beginning to pay more attention to the ways in which health is influenced by mental and emotional states. Meditation also helps insomnia. In fact, people who have difficulty falling asleep can usually fall asleep in about 15 minutes when they practice meditation. If you need help, meditation tapes and cassettes are available. Ask your doctor about these.

Visualization is a technique first used by a radiation oncologist[225] to help patients help themselves by changing their lifestyle either to eliminate stressful situations or to reduce them. Part of visualization is maintaining a positive attitude and refusing to allow negative feelings to interfere with one's return to health. For more information on visualization, consult your doctor.

PROSTHESIS OR RECONSTRUCTION

A few ounces of foam rubber can never replace a breast, or help a woman live with the fact that she has had cancer. Still, for many women, prostheses or external breast forms are a sensible, accepted alternative to further surgery. These forms can make most women look normal and feel physically and emotionally complete even in the most revealing clothes. Most large department stores and a number of specialty shops carry many wardrobe items for the mastectomy patient. Some of these shops are run by women who have had the operation themselves and understand the problems.

Many health insurance plans will pay for breast prostheses. However, some women prefer to use inexpensive, homemade breast forms. One patient of mine told me that she had tried several prostheses, but found the one she made herself worked best and looked the most natural. Patients of mine have used pantyhose, socks, cotton and other available material as fillers. Others found that by wearing loose-fitting, but stylish clothing they could present a perfectly normal appearance. More important, however, individuals who are able to adjust their attitudes as well as their lifestyles respond well to recovery and have fewer emotional problems.

My advice to any woman who has had a mastectomy is not to isolate herself from others. If you have a hobby, check to see if your local college or night school offers courses in the subject. Investigate social groups that are organized by churches, temples, or other private organizations. Make a real effort to broaden your social contacts. If you always eat at home or watch TV alone, occasionally try going out to a movie or eating at a restaurant with friends.

Invariably the woman who has had a breast removed, particularly those who are unmarried or divorced, will at least consider reconstruction. There are several types of operations using implants or other methods (see chapter 19, Breast Reconstruction After Mastectomy), but they are all expensive and not without risks. For the woman who is highly motivated, breast reconstruction can be a blessing.

There is no reason to run away from cancer or avoid treatment. In many instances cancer can be completely cured, and the lives of some famous women attest to this fact: Julia Child, Shirley Temple Black, Betty Rollin,[226] Betty Ford, Happy Rockefeller, and Nancy Reagan. They all continue to be active and productive, many years after their diagnosis and treatment.

THE QUALITY OF LIFE

If we talk about the quality of life of the breast cancer patient, we have to discuss all patients afflicted with the disease. Not all patients have tiny breast cancers and not all treatments are successful. Nor do all patients do well following a mastectomy, or lumpectomy with radiation treatment. Some women develop recurrent cancer, cancer that has spread to different anatomical areas. It is the job of the breast cancer specialist dealing with recurrent breast cancer to think about how to palliate these women and assist them in reconstructing a life that they believe is worth continuing.

Quality of survival[227] is determined by how a patient lives and survives after they develop a disease and are treated. The concept itself demands open discussion and debate, for if a patient does not return to work, or resume normal body functions and social communication with her family, friends, and the outside world, she does not have a good quality of survival. There are moral, ethical, and economic questions that must be considered, not only by the breast cancer patient and her family, but by all patients who have a serious disease.

Whether the woman with breast cancer has a quality of survival that she can be proud of depends not only on the individual herself, but the doctor treating her, the response of her family to her emotional needs, and on the levels of communication used in working out the trauma associated with the disease.

There are many questions: how does one define quality of survival, since each survivor may have different values and goals in life? How does the patient feel about her treatment? Is she healthy? The stage of her disease is important when answering this question, since the surgery, radiation, or chemotherapy treatment, or combinations thereof, are usually more aggressive for the serious breast tumor.

If the disease has spread to her regional nodes (lymph glands) or there is systemic spread (bones, lungs, liver, brain) chemotherapy is often the recommended treatment. Will she accept this with optimism, or will she be depressed and limited in her ability to return to work or conduct her usual activities?

Studies have been done comparing endocrine (hormonal) and cyto-toxic (chemo) therapy in women with advanced breast cancer. If the patients see their tumors responding to treatment, they are better able to tolerate the toxic side effects of the chemotherapy. However, if there is no response, the treatment's toxicity becomes unbearable. Some patients cannot tolerate the nausea, vomiting, or loss of hair that often occurs with these treatments and will not continue with the chemotherapy protocols (treatment).

With improved treatments providing better cure rates for breast cancer and increased length of survival, how do patients do in terms of quality of life after mastectomy or other treatment?

My research confirms the fact that too much emphasis has been placed on cancer as an enigma, and that the quality of survival depends to a great degree upon what has been called the "hopelessness potential"—a psychological scale that measures how much control women felt they had over their lives, futures, and the state of their health. A disproportionate number of breast cancer patients seem to live in an emotional slump—often feeling helpless, worried, and pessimistic. They tend to repress their anger but accept their depression. They ignore their achievements but embrace their failures.

For a long time, however, these observations were *merely* observations, informal suspicions that a person's mental state might somehow play a role in the treatment of cancer. It wasn't until the latter half of this century that these suspicions began to harden into scientific theory. The doctors at several university hospitals evaluated women who had to undergo biopsies for breast lumps for signs of depression and other emotional disorders.

The results were sobering. Women who had been diagnosed with depression prior to their breast cancer diagnosis had an increased death rate from cancer—twice as high as the rate in the general population. Other risk factors—such as obesity or stress—were taken into account in these investigations. However, it was concluded that depression alone was a critical factor in the patient's length of survival. Doctors were not looking for depression per se, but for traumatic events that had preceded the development of the disease or followed its treatment.

Why should what goes on in our minds be expressed in our cells? The answer may be in the immune system. In the healthiest person, scattered cancer cells may occasionally appear and begin to multiply. When the immune system is functioning as it should, white blood cells exterminate the rogue malignancies. If, however, the immune system falters—responds too late or too listlessly—cancer may have a chance to take hold.

Skeptics question the reliability of these findings. Doctors who support this type of research admit that diagnosing emotional conditions and establishing their relationship to physical health is an imprecise science at best. Does depression really *precede* cancer, or does cancer—even before it's discovered—wrack the body so that one begins to feel defeated and depressed without knowing why? Do those who interview women after a biopsy for breast cancer get a true picture of the woman's feelings of hope or hopelessness?

My own feeling is that a chronically repressed or depressed temperament is a cancer signpost, not a cancer sentence. Until recently most women *feared* that mastectomy was the usual treatment for breast cancer and that the disease was incurable. This is completely wrong. More and more women are now preserving their breast and many are being cured. Fewer and fewer women are having mastectomies. There are, indeed, reasons for regarding cancer as a serious enemy. These are not reasons for anxiety or depression. Quite the contrary—the killer has not been isolated and destroyed, but it is being cornered. To vanquish it from our bodies and our society will take a strong heart and unwavering conviction.

No longer should any woman feel that she must lose a breast to cancer. If that does become necessary, she should know that her life can still be a long and happy one. She has no reason to believe that she can't have children, or that she won't be around to raise the ones she does have.

Those patients who resume their household duties or return to work without turning inward to dwell on their wound showed more optimism about their lives. In my opinion, their willingness to fight had a beneficial effect on their immune system that equaled the power of anticancer drugs. They never felt abandoned, even when there was a recurrence, and their ability to face adversity was crucial to their continued survival.

SUMMARY

No one benefits from studies that suggest, even obliquely, that cancer patients somehow brought their illness on themselves. But emotions can play an important part in each phase of cancer, from early detection, to treatment and recovery. Those who maintain a positive emotional vigil have been shown to have high cure rates and successful rehabilitation. Nowhere is psychology as important as in the treatment of cancer, with all its inchoate fears. And women can, with a little assistance, learn to fight and conquer these fears.

QUESTIONS

Q. *Should the patient be told all the details of their cancer or spread of their cancer? Should they be told the truth?*

A. I think you have to listen to the patient. They will often tell you how much or how little and how often they want to talk about their diagnosis and future. The doctor's answers to the patient's questions should be candid and unembellished. I feel the patient should be told the truth. Most of the time this helps maintain a good healthy doctor/patient relationship. If the patient, at some point, finds that the doctor kept some facts regarding her diagnosis from her, she may not trust the doctor in the future.

Q. *What do you tell a woman who must undergo a mastectomy?*

A. First I tell her that saving her life is more important than saving her breast. It is then possible to discuss the type of surgery, how it may affect breast reconstruction, and similar patients' results. If the woman is married, it helps to have her husband present at this time so that emotional rehabilitation can begin prior to surgery.

Q. *What do you tell a woman who has a lumpectomy, axillary dissection, and radiation therapy?*

A. I tell her that she is fortunate that she has a minimal cancer and has the option of breast conservation surgery. I also tell her that it may be more difficult to monitor her for local recurrence after radiation therapy and that there can be some delayed problems from radiation.

Q. *What do you tell a woman who had a mastectomy followed by breast reconstruction?*

A. That it will be more difficult to monitor the mastectomy site, since a silicone gel prosthesis will be placed over the chest wall defect.

Q. *Is it natural to be depressed after a mastectomy?*

A. Of course. What isn't natural is to be depressed months and months later, or to isolate oneself from normal social contacts because of the operation. Those patients who do the best usually adjust immediately or within a short period of time. Both doctor and family can be supportive to ease this transition.

Q. *How can a husband help the mastectomy patient?*

A. By being loving and understanding of the operation and consistently warm and forthright in his actions. Many husbands are fearful of doing or saying the wrong thing and this can appear to be rejection when it really is not. He can also be sensitive to any clues his wife gives to how she feels.

Q. *Do you prescribe tranquilizers or other drugs?*

A. It depends on the circumstances. There's no reason not to if the patient has taken such medications in the past, or is anxious or in pain. Each case has to be treated individually and, in some instances, I recommend psychological counseling.

Q. *Why is there such a preoccupation with breasts in our society?*

A. Today's modern fashions contribute to this. Perhaps if women wore *saris* as they do in India, or slit skirts, as in the Far East, there would not be so much emphasis on a woman's breasts. Women themselves are not blameless in this preoccupation as they act according to what fashion demands.

Q. *What can you tell children about breast cancer?*

A. Not much, if they are young. The word cancer itself scares most children, as it does adults, and children may not be old enough to cope with the knowledge. Older children can cope better and should be told about the operation and what it means. In my experience they are often supportive.

Q. *Why do you emphasize the psychology of cancer?*

A. We have gone about as far as possible in surgical treatment and we tend to ignore the rehabilitation of breast cancer patients. Emotions can play an important role in the recovery process and even help prevent recurrence. This, and current experiments with anticancer drugs, are perhaps the most exciting areas of research at the present time.

Q. *What do you mean by quality of survival?*

A. The way the patient adjusts to her treatment and how it affects her future. It's not possible to predict how an individual will respond, but a doctor can offer practical advice and guidance based on the experiences of other women who have had breast cancer.

Q. *Can anything be done for the woman with advanced breast cancer?*

A. There are a number of promising anticancer drugs that work on the cancer cell and the immune system to prevent spread of the cancer. Scientists are working to lessen their side-effects to make such treatments more bearable.

Q. *What do you tell the woman with advanced cancer who has no chance of survival?*

A. Despite the moral, ethical, and economic questions of treating terminal patients, my feeling is that every patient should have the right to seek and obtain treatment, even if it is only palliative. She should not be abandoned to hopelessness. She should be assured that attempts will be made to help her and to relieve her pain.

Q. *Why do you feel that way?*

A. We are transplanting organs and making artificial ones every day for patients who would otherwise die. New drugs are also being found for diseases once thought incurable. There is no reason why one or more cures couldn't be found for cancer of the breast. Hope, not despair, should guide the choice of each patient with cancer.

Q. *How do you feel about cancer insurance?*

A. It is a good idea for the high-risk patient. Some two million policies are sold each year. The reason is that, per patient, the total medical cost for treating some breast cancers can be more than $200,000. Whether cancer insurance actually provides adequate financial protection is questionable. Some policies pay only one-third of hospital costs. Others will not cover complications, or impose a time limit after a cancer is first diagnosed. An alternative might be an "excess major medical rider" to an existing health insurance policy, such as catastrophic insurance.

25

The Outlook for the Future

Rapid progress has occurred in breast cancer research and treatment since the publication of *Breast Care Options* in 1986. Many investigative areas have contributed to the advancement of detection and treatment. The five-year survival rate is now 74 percent. New, innovative techniques are supplementing older methods. National Cancer Institute endeavors are gathering statistics which are helping to determine the best ways to treat breast cancer.

Much of what we know about breast cancer seems intractable, but now even the entrenched radical mastectomy has given way to many new breast care options that can save lives and, in selected cases, preserve the breast. Researchers in many fields, not just oncology, have contributed to the progress in earlier detection (mammography, ultrasound, magnetic resonance imaging). When breast cancer is detected when it is small, treatment is usually less radical.

Breast self-examination is still important but mammography is playing an increasing role in the detection of breast cancer. Fifty percent of the breast cancer patients I see in my office have tumors detected by mammography. This means that more breast cancers are being detected when they are small; survival rates should therefore increase.

Mammography is also detecting an increasing number of simultaneous bilateral breast cancers, in which x-rays show cancer in both breasts at the same time. This discovery has increased the controversy over whether breast cancer is a systemic disease from the onset.

If breast cancer is a systemic disease, new methods of controlling it can be developed. Ten years ago, this view would have been ridiculed and few dared to challenge the prevailing wisdom. But the recent alert by the National Cancer Institute recommending that chemotherapy should be given to all breast cancer patients if the nodes (glands) in the armpit are not involved suggests that some leading scientists suspect that breast cancer is definitely a systemic disease.

However, node–negative patients present a unique situation because not all the facts are in. It would be extremely costly to give chemotherapy for six months to all patients with small cancers. The increased benefit to the patients is small and the long-term morbidity and mortality is unpredictable.

Just what does a woman do if she develops a suspicious breast lump? What are some of the breast care options for the 1990's? Thousands of women are learning that breast cancer need not be the dreadful, mutilating killer it has been in the past. Cancer management is becoming increasingly individualized, both in respect to diagnostic procedures and treatment. Early detection is now followed by a precise staging of the disease and often more than one method of therapy is used.

With medical progress producing better cure rates and longer survival, the focus is shifting toward the woman's psychological needs. Investigators are studying the patient's and family's reactions to the disease, sexual concerns, employment and insurance needs, and specific ways to provide support.

Many breast cancer patients become depressed when they learn they have cancer. New drugs such as Prozac (an antidepressant) and other medications have been developed. Some say Prozac is the miracle drug to help alleviate the depression that numerous breast cancer patients experience.

There are five million Americans alive today who have a history of cancer, and three million of those were diagnosed five or more years ago. Most can be considered cured. That is, they have no evidence of the disease and have the same life expectancy as a person who never had cancer. Others can expect to be saved by earlier diagnosis and prompt treatment. For localized noninvasive (in situ) breast cancer, the survival rate approaches 100 percent. The survival rates for all forms of cancer are on the increase, except for lung cancer.

What this means is that progress is being made. In the future, the search will continue for newer and better ways to treat or prevent the disease.

BENEFITS OF EARLY DETECTION

The time to detect cancer is early, when it is emminently treatable. In their joint Breast Cancer Detection Demonstration Program, the American Cancer Society and National Cancer Institute found that mammography (low-dose x-ray examination) could find cancers so small they could not be felt by even the most experienced examiner. Other experiments using sound waves, infrared heat patterns, computers, and electromagnets offer the hope that one day even the smallest cancers will be identified and treated before they get out of control.

Research is also being directed toward other detection devices that do not use radiation at all. The same high-energy sound waves used to destroy kidney stones, for example, may prove to be a new way to detect and treat breast cancer. Techniques such as thermography (infrared heat patterns) and computerized tomography (CT scans) to show a tumor's shape and location more accurately are being studied for their possible effectiveness and applications.

But of all the diagnostic newcomers, perhaps the most revolutionary is magnetic resonance imaging (MRI), which uses a huge electromagnet to detect tumors by sensing the vibrations of the different atoms in the body. It also permits detailed study of cell physiology, which can help us determine just why the cancer cell goes haywire and how the body's immune system does and does not react to it. Recent studies of proteins in the blood are providing doctors with new methods in detecting early breast cancers. The nature and role of growth factors and a tumor's receptors in the breast have also been more clearly defined. Research scientists are now finding abnormalities in specific genes that may be present in breast cancer specimens. As we gain greater knowledge of the genetic changes that play a role in cancer cell growth we should be able to design new therapeutic strategies to forestall or eradicate that growth.

It's obvious that we are making progress, but you, as a patient, can help also. Clearly, thousands of lives could be saved each year through early detection, not only of breast cancer, but cancers of the cervix, uterus, and colon, which offer the greatest opportunity for treatment and cure. For this reason, it's most important for women to practice monthly breast self-examination, have mammograms or other medical tests, and become familiar with the guidelines for the early detection of cancer.

THE FUTURE OF BREAST SURGERY

The surgical treatment of breast cancer has undergone dramatic changes during the past 100 years. Radical treatment of breast cancer is infrequent (3 percent) and surgical techniques to save the breast are now in vogue since survival results are similar.

Improvements in early detection and staging of the disease have made limited surgery possible in the management of tiny cancers. This means that many patients have been able to retain all or part of their breast. For others, advances in reconstructive surgery, using skin-muscle grafts or implants, have become important choices for women who have had a mastectomy.

Surgical equipment is also being improved. A surgical tool that can be harnessed to microwaves to "cook" or cauterize wounds at the same moment an incision is made, has been a promising innovation. This technique has the advantage of closing the blood vessels and lymphatics by coagulation at the moment the tissue is cut. A laser scalpel is also being used to treat areas in the body to prevent damage to surrounding healthy tissue. Freezing tumors with extreme cold (cryosurgery) is another method of destroying tumors.

All women should realize, however, that conservative or limited surgery (lumpectomy or quadrectomy) will not become the treatment of choice for all breast cancers even in the future, because a significant number of breast cancers are still detected in the advanced stage, when limited surgery is neither effective nor practical. This may change as more tumors are detected in the earlier noninvasive stage and we learn more about the long-term results of such conservation operations. Right now, limited surgery followed by radiation therapy is competing with modified mastectomy as the treatment of choice.

RADIATION

Diagnostic methods, using new radiation techniques, have made a tremendous advance during the past decade. I've mentioned that there has been a drastic reduction in x-ray exposure through development of special mammographic films and the grid technique. When mammography was first introduced, the breast tumor patient was exposed to excessive and therefore dangerous amounts of radiation (as much as 15 rads for one diagnostic procedure). Today, that same procedure can be done with three-tenths of a rad exposure to the breast. For a woman over 50 years of age, the risk is minimal. For a woman under 30 years of age, the risk is still present and precautions should be taken.

Radiation treatment methods for breast cancer have become more sophisticated during the past decade. Computer-controlled x-ray machines are more precise in treating the affected area and reducing the damage to the surrounding healthy tissue.

Intraoperative radiation is being studied as a way to give x-ray treatment at the time of surgery for breast cancer and colon cancer, the idea being to eliminate residual cancer cells. There's little evidence, however, that such treatment, during or following limited surgery, (lumpectomy, for example) works effectively on every patient.

For patients who do undergo radiation therapy, frequent scanning by computerized tomography may enable the radiologist to pinpoint the tumor and administer radiation more accurately, sparing normal tissue. This is the subject of several recent studies and the results are being put into clinical use at many large hospitals. Elsewhere, researchers are trying to develop a special bra that contains sensors to pick up "hot spots" in breast tissue that could signal a malignancy. Radioactive implants have also been used in women recovering from a lumpectomy to destroy any residual cancer cells.

Scientists are still looking for the diagnostic instrument that will not expose the body to ionizing radiation. The use of magnetic resonance imaging may eventually be that instrument. It can outline blood vessels such as the large arteries in the neck (carotids) without using invasive catheters and dyes to determine if there is an arteriosclerotic plaque obstructing the blood vessel.

The horizons are unlimited for innovative new techniques and rapid progress is being made in breast cancer research. There is *hope*.

CHEMOTHERAPY

Radical surgery and radical radiation treatment can go just so far in trying to eliminate cancer. Surgery and radiation treat localized cancer, at a specific anatomical site. Chemotherapy is the use of drugs that are

212 • *Breast Care Options for the 1990's*

injected or given in pill form, to reach and destroy cancer cells through the bloodstream or lymphatics. Cancer cells may spread to distant areas of the body (metastasize), and represent an added threat to the host.

Chemotherapy still has not been completely successful in preventing the recurrence or spread of breast cancer, but it has been useful in interfering with the rapid cell division and growth of the cancer cell. Today, many patients with breast cancer are being treated successfully with combination chemotherapy (cytotoxic drugs and hormones) to shrink advanced tumors or induce a remission.

The next step is to see if these and other agents can reduce cancer in high-risk patients by interrupting the process in which different kinds of substances, known as initiators and promoters, cause the cancer to develop and spread. Unusual infections, common in cancer patients, may also be better controlled by new antibiotic treatment and antibodies.

Why do some patients object to chemotherapy? The chief reason is that when large amounts of toxic chemotherapeutic agents are used, the bone marrow, which produces all blood cells, is destroyed. Large doses of chemotherapy and radiation sometimes destroy the tumor, but in the process of doing so also destroy the host.

A new costly but effective method has been developed to prevent this from happening. It is called autologous marrow transplant. Doctors remove part of the patient's bone marrow before the patient receives massive doses of chemotherapy to knock out the tumor. The preserved marrow is then returned to make new cells and thereby speed the patient's recovery. It has worked for lymphomas and leukemias and looks like it might work for breast cancer patients.

What do patients receiving chemotherapy object to most? Patients have stated that the worst thing is the horrible nausea and vomiting. Some say they will never take chemotherapy again. Fortunately, progress is being made. It's felt that the symptoms that cause nausea and vomiting are due to the chemotherapeutic agents releasing serotonin, a neurotransmitter, into the gastrointestinal tract. New antiemetic drugs have been developed which are serotonin antagonists, preventing nausea and vomiting by blocking serotonin production in the bowel and the brain and thereby stopping the nerve impulses that cause vomiting. It seems to be working and is a tremendous boon to chemotherapy patients.

The use of chemotherapy infusion pumps that administer chemotherapy over a long period of time has also proved helpful. Studies indicate that successful chemotherapy may be best achieved by timing the introduction of drugs to the patient at a time when they can be tolerated better. About 50 or more drugs have been found effective against cancer, and others that hold promise are being tested.

IMMUNOTHERAPY

We've seen that surgery, chemotherapy, and radiation, or a combination of the three, have failed so far to come up with a total cure for breast cancer.

I have always thought the immune system and how it works is the most important aspect in controlling breast cancer. Anyone who has treated large numbers of breast cancer patients realizes how variable the individual's bodily response is. Some patients have a small breast cancer and no matter how you treat them, the cancer is relentless and the patient succumbs in a short period of time. Others have larger, advanced cancers and yet their alarm system (immune system) is able to respond and they live a useful and healthy life.

The importance of the immune system is dramatically portrayed in the high incidence of cancer in patients who have had liver transplants. When a patient undergoes an organ transplant, the immune system lights up and tries to reject the foreign tissue. To prevent rejection, immunosuppressive drugs such as Cyclosporin are given for prolonged periods of time. When the immune system is suppressed for long periods of time, the patient is at great risk for getting cancer, and that's often exactly what happens. Dr. Thomas Starzl, Professor of Surgery at the University of Pittsburgh, observed that liver transplant patients had a cancer incidence ten times that of the normal population.

Scientists have just started to unlock the method by which the immune system functions. Research in major medical centers is identifying patients who are at high risk for developing breast cancer. Autologous skin tests to determine how capable a patient's immune system is of fighting an invading cancer are being developed. If a patient's immune system is poor, an aggressive treatment regimen can then be instituted.

I predict that future treatment methods will develop once we isolate the initiating factor in breast cancer (virus, chemicals, hormones, or their combinations). We should be able to identify the cell components that react to fight the cancer. We should then be able to grow these agents in genetic factories and use them to enhance the body's immune system response. The possibility of developing a vaccine is not as far-fetched as some people think, particularly for those individuals in the high-risk group.

Cancer researchers have already developed ways to strengthen the immune system through experiments in which more natural killer cells are put into action against some cancers. Lymphokines, a type of white blood cell, are produced in response to an attack of cancer cells on the human body. They go around alerting the immune system to "light up" and fight the invaders. We are just beginning to learn more about lymphokines and tumor necrosis factors, which destroy cancer cells but leave normal cells untouched. As we learn more, we will be able to manipulate them better, and their use will become more valuable.

CAN CANCER BE PREVENTED?

Chemoprevention studies of agents like synthetic retinoids (cousins of vitamin A), beta-carotene, folic acid, and other vitamins and minerals are being undertaken to see if they can prevent cancer. Studies of dietary intervention are exploring the effect of low-fat diets on women with breast cancer. As the risk for breast, uterine, and colon cancers increases for obese women, this is an area worthy of investigation.

Extensive research is underway to evaluate and clarify the role of diet and nutrition in the development of cancer. At this point, no direct cause-and-effect relationship has been proven, though several studies show that some foods may increase or decrease the risks for certain types of cancer. Evidence indicates that women might reduce their breast cancer risk by eating more cruciferous vegetables (cabbage, broccoli), foods rich in vitamin A and C (carrots, oranges), and low-fat acidophilus milk, which may prevent breast cancer by limiting estrogen circulation and carcinogen-generating enzymes.

Unproven methods of cancer prevention or treatment are bound to surface in the future, and the findings of the research done on them should be evaluated carefully by patients and doctors alike. A list of ingredients is mandatory on most food and drug products, so the best advice is to read all the labeling carefully and make an informed decision.

SUMMARY

Until 100 years ago, medicine was practiced as an imprecise art: the physician used his eyes, ears, and hands to accumulate data and information.

Today, with sophisticated machines, we are able to penetrate the human body and outline its anatomical structures. X-ray machines, CT scans (computed axial tomography) and ultrasound (the use of sound waves) and magnetic resonance imaging machines visualize preselected parts of the human body. Using computer reconstruction techniques, we are able to get clearer pictures. Magnetic resonance imaging, using a giant magnet, is now imaging the cell structure itself and in the near future should be able to tell us about the many complicated factors that play a role in producing cancer.

Never before has so much money, effort and research been mobilized to combat this powerful foe called cancer. With the successful treatment of localized, noninvasive breast cancer now approaching 100 percent, overall cure rates are moving upward with heart-lifting speed. Medical science alone cannot conquer cancer, and my advice is to take steps now to outwit and avoid cancer as you would any other danger lurking about.

26
An Attempt to Define Cancer

Cancer was named by Hippocrates,[228,229,230,231,232,233] the father of medicine. The Greek word is *karkinos*, or crab, so named because of the pincer-like projections he noticed when examining women with breast cancer. A disease which today would be called cancer was described and written about by the Egyptians 3,000 years before the birth of Christ.[234] Of course, the disease they described was always fatal. As a result, doctors in ancient times thought cancer incurable.

There have been two main concepts argued about for centuries as to how breast cancer starts, and the controversy still lives.

The first concept was that breast cancer is a systemic disease from its onset. This concept was proposed as early as the second century by Galen[235] (131–203 A.D.). He attributed cancer to an excess of bile distributed throughout the body. In other words, the cancer was in all the tissues and was believed to have a genetic origin.

In the 18th century (1757), a French surgeon, Henry Francois Le Dran,[236] advanced the theory that cancer began in its earliest stages as a local disease—if treated properly it could be cured. If not, it would spread first by lymphatics to regional nodes and subsequently would enter the general circulation. This was the first challenge to the systemic theory of breast cancer.

In the 19th century, the discovery of the microscope was a giant step in helping to understand just what cancer was. Now the cancerous tissue could be sectioned, stained, and the cells analyzed under the microscope. The microscope opened new avenues of research.

In 1858, Virchow[237] proposed that any normal cell can become a cancer cell as a result of irritation. Was he talking about environmental hazards affecting the normal cell, or internal sources of irritation? We are left to wonder.

In 1867, Charles H. Moore,[238] at the Middlesex Hospital of London, readvocated the idea of breast cancer originating locally. He observed that recurrences after limited operations for breast cancer were generally near the scar. He concluded that surgical failure was due not to systemic spread but to failure of the surgeon to remove all local extensions of disease.

It soon became apparent that the cancer cell could spread (metastasize) outside the local area and cause the death of the host. The realization that surgical failures are actually due to tumor spread (metastases) was the most important factor that led to the present-day era of systemic chemotherapy.

It is still not known why certain women get breast cancer and others do not. Recent research suggests that genetics, lifestyles, and environmental factors are interlocked in their influence. If breast cancer exists in your family tree, you are at greater risk to get it. Recent studies show that women who eat a diet rich in fatty foods and are obese are more prone to getting breast cancer. Hormones and stress also are causative factors.

WHAT IS A CANCER CELL?

What we do know is that cancer is a large group of diseases characterized by uncontrolled growth and spread of abnormal or malignant cells. The human body is made up of millions of cells that combine to form tissues and organs with specific functions, enabling the organism to survive and adapt to a changing environment. The normal healthy cell has a specific site it functions at. It requires water, food, and oxygen to survive and is capable of duplication and reproduction.

The cancer cell varies from the normal healthy cell. It has a marked diversity in regard to reproduction and morphology. The cell surface, or membrane, is different; it is able to invade tissues and organs and destroy them. It has abnormal growth rates and can spread to distant organs, where it attaches itself to form new cancers.

Both the normal cell and the cancer cell have a control mechanism, or nucleus, inside the cell. The cancer cell is different in that it is able to multiply more rapidly. Its nucleus is often divided or in the process of dividing. If there are many abnormal cells like this seen under the microscope, the diagnosis of cancer is made.

What causes the normal cell to become a cancer cell and go haywire is still unknown. Is it due to a virus? If so, how does the virus penetrate the normal cell membrane and get at the nucleus, which controls the cell's action?

Or is a cell cancerous from the beginning? Is it a mutant that has been developed by environmental effects upon the cell, such as chemicals, nutrients, or adverse oxygenation effects?

We know that the cell has a membrane and that nutrients and chemicals diffuse in and out of the cell through the membrane. The cancer cell interacts with the normal healthy cell and therefore, in order to penetrate or spread, the cell membrane is important. The ability of the cancer cell membrane to stick to a blood vessel wall determines the capability of the cancer cell to metastasize, or spread.

Not all cancer cells metastasize. Why some spread and others do not is difficult to determine. When cancer does spread, its cells, or clumps of cells, can break off (tumor emboli) and get into the lymphatics (nodes or glands) or into the bloodstream.

As a tumor grows, not all its cells are actively dividing. As the tumor continues to grow and get larger, the percentage of actively dividing cells may decrease. This may be due to blood supply or other factors, such as hormones, or the body's own defense mechanism attempting to slow down the growth of the tumor.

Tumors have a measurable rate of growth. This is called the doubling time of the tumor. It is the time the cancer cell takes to reproduce itself. The range of doubling time can vary immensely—from one week to two years or much longer. For example, the typical breast cancer usually takes two years to reach one-half inch and eight years to grow big enough to be detected.

THE WAY CANCER SPREADS

Local Invasion

Cancer cells can invade and destroy local tissues. If local invasion occurs and the cancer is in an area of the body that can be surgically removed without endangering the patient, surgery can control the cancer. Radiation can control the smaller cancers if distant spread has not occurred.

An example of a tumor that invades locally is a skin cancer (basal cell) that often occurs on the exposed areas of the body and is related to prolonged exposure to sunlight (radiation). Excellent treatment results can be attained by surgery or radiation.

However, in contrast to skin cancers, other local cancer invasions can be lethal if the tumor develops in an area of the body that cannot be easily resected surgically or treated by other methods. For example, esophageal cancer (the esophagus is the feeding tube from the mouth to the stomach) is located in an area of the body that cannot easily be removed. The heart and breathing tubes that go to the lungs are right next to the esophagus, making it more difficult to treat this area.

Certain brain tumors are another example of how local invasion can destroy the host and because of their location they rarely spread outside of the skull. These tumors are very difficult to treat.

Metastases

If the cancer specialist could prevent metastases from occurring, most cancers could be cured by controlling the primary tumor if it occurs at a site that can be adequately treated. Once the cell or cells have broken off from the primary tumor, the cells flow to glands or distant organs usually through lymphatics or vascular channels. Osmotic pressures or mobility of the cells themselves aid the flow.

The cancer cells' ability to form a clump of cells and metastasize to a distant site has something to do with the complex mechanism of blood clotting. It is also necessary that a certain concentration of cancer cells be present in order to get a take (metastases) at a distant site. It has been known for years that migratory thrombophlebitis can be associated with diffuse overwhelming cancer (pancreatic cancer, for instance).

The mechanism by which blood clots—or does not clot—when patients have cancer is unclear. The hypercoagulable state, or increased tendency to clot, associated with cancer probably has something to do with thrombin (an enzyme that participates in the blood clotting) and the venous vessel wall and breakdown products of the necrotic tumor.

Migratory thrombophlebitis is resistant to routine anticoagulant therapy and may appear months or years before cancer develops. The human body's mechanism by which blood remains liquid is unclear. There are many factors in the vascular system that prevent blood from clotting, such as fibrinolytic enzymes.

Attempts have been made to prevent metastases by giving blood thinners such as heparin and dicumerol and this has been successful in preventing metastases in laboratory experiments. It has not been successful in humans.

Cancer cells have other interesting characteristics which should be mentioned in regard to metastasis. Once the clump of cancer cells or metastasis has anchored at a distant site (usually in the capillary beds) neovascularization of the tumor occurs. By neovascularization, I mean that new blood vessels grow as the tumor gets larger. The rate of growth of the lining of the blood vessels feeding the tumor (the endothelium) might have something to do with the actual size of the tumor.

The properties of the vessel wall (endothelium) are extremely important, for if the vessel wall is damaged, the clotting mechanism (coagulation process) goes on more rapidly, particularly in the small vessels on the surface, or smaller peripheral vessels in organs. It is here that the rate of flow is lower and the exchange of nutrients and chemicals through cell membranes occurs.

Not all cancer cells or clumps of cells that break off from the primary tumor are capable of taking hold at the distant site. In fact, very few actually survive. This may be related to their inability to attach to the vessel, or to the cohesiveness of the cancer cell, or to the host's resistance.

Once the cancer cells get free, the body's immune mechanism comes into play. The ability of one human body to destroy circulating cancer cells and another to allow it to take, or metastasize, relates to the immune mechanism.

Immune mechanism

The immune mechanism works in several different ways, not all of which are fully understood. Basically, certain types of white blood cells are alerted to the presence of invading cancer cells and form antibodies to fight and destroy the invaders. This can be seen graphically in the rejection of donor tissue or organs during transplant operations, and is the subject of a lot of research.

Manmade antibodies such as hybridomas (antibody factories), and specific monoclonal antibodies that will only recognize cancer cells can be produced and used to fight the disease. Monoclonal antibodies already have been used to deliver drugs directly to tumors, killing them but sparing healthy tissue. Gene splicing has produced interferon, which may ultimately be valued not so much for itself, as for its role in heralding a whole new class of compounds called "biologic response modifiers," which will fight cancer by stimulating the body's immune system.

As we increase our knowledge of the immune system, we can expect genetic engineering endeavors to find other ways to fight cancer. Investigators are already looking for ways to detect cancer earlier by tracing a cell's biochemical markers. They are exploring evidence that certain organs or parts of the body tend to be more involved than others because of a breakdown in the individual's immune system. They're testing the hypothesis that certain chemicals or environments enhance the body's receptivity to cancer.

Epidemiologists know, for example, that cancer affects people in some parts of the world more than others and that breast cancer is more common in obese women who eat fatty foods than in thinner women whose diet is low in fat and high in protein. They point to the high incidence of cervical cancer among women who are sexually active, and to the increased rates of lung cancer among women smokers. Other clues being pursued by researchers suggest certain lifestyles serve as defense mechanisms against cancer.

Fortunately, cancer is not contagious. Or is it? Recently, the disease entity AIDS, which can be transmitted sexually or through the blood, was found to produce Kaposi's sarcoma, a form of cancer. It is perhaps one of the few types of cancers that can be transmitted by a virus. Yet virtually all cancers are not contagious.

Selection of site of metastases

There also seems to be a selective process by cancer cells as to where they live and grow. This concept was set forth by Steven Paget in 1889. He believed in the theory of "seed and soil"—that cancer cells lodge and grow selectively at favorable locations.

Specific organs seem to be the most common sites of metastases, and these sites can be predicted in certain cancers. Other organs are less often involved with metastatic disease, bringing us to the question: is the tissue in certain areas not fertile for the cancer seed to grow? Or does that organ contain anticancer substances? An example is the spleen, which is not often involved with metastatic cancer and yet if an overwhelming infection in the body occurs, the spleen frequently shows evidence of the infection. How often has one seen the bones of the hands or feet involved with metastatic cancer? Yet in breast cancer the other bones of the body are frequently involved. When a patient gets more than one cancer there seems to be a specific site at which the second cancer will develop.[129]

Factors that produce cancers

The exogenous factors that produce cancer are too numerous to mention. An important one we see in our daily lives is radiation from the sun, which can produce skin cancers, such as basal cell cancer. Radiation probably plays a role in activating the lethal pigmented melanoma of the skin. Incriminating evidence that viruses are involved appears every day in research.

The acquired immune deficiency syndrome (AIDS), still seen predominantly in male homosexuals, and can be transmitted by blood, is known to produce cancerous tumors known as Kaposi's sarcoma, in all likelihood caused by a virus. This disease has prompted the scientific community to study the role of viral infections in relation to causative factors, the immune system and the production of a deadly cancer.

Other viruses too have been identified as factors in precancerous and invasive cancers of the cervix. These too may be sexually transmitted.

A human papillomavirus (HPU) has been isolated and can produce tumors of the esophagus. It also has been linked to squamous cell cancer in other body areas. This virus, which is acquired either congenitally or through sexual transmission, may be increasing because of the prevalence of oral-genital sexual intercourse.

The food we eat and the water we drink are extremely important factors to consider. The benefits of natural foods, citrus fruits, and foods with high concentrations of vitamins A and C have been written about extensively. Additives to preserve food, as well as artificial colorings or flavorings, have been linked to cancer.

Pesticides and chemical wastes from industrial plants that get into our drinking water can trigger cancer and workers in asbestos plants who were not properly protected invariably developed debilitating lung disease and cancer. So, while you can't live in a hermetically sealed home, you can stay informed of outside cancer-causing agents and be on guard against them.

DOES AGE PLAY A ROLE IN PRODUCING CANCER?

As the body ages and its parts start to wear out, is the immune response capable of handling an invasion by cancer? Only a small number of cancers occur in the younger age group and many of these may be related to genetic factors. But the stress of living in today's society takes its toll and contributes to the aging process, and, as stated herein, stress and the immune system are interrelated.

Most cancers occur in the fourth, fifth, and sixth decades of life. Age certainly is a factor in the development of breast cancer. In my practice, 90 percent of breast cancers developed after the age of 38 years. Only 10 percent occurred before. Most breast cancers develop during or shortly after menopause. This is most likely because with the aging process, the body's tissues and cells start to wear out, and women become more susceptible to cancer at that time.

As researchers unlock the mechanisms of the immune system, we should be able to find the key to a cure for breast cancer in the future.

SUMMARY

Trying to define how cancer develops is an insurmountable problem at the present time, although great progress is being made.

Eminent scientists have difficulty explaining the complex nature of the cancer cell. Recent research suggests that cancer can be related to genetic defects, and the environment that we live in may play an important role in lighting the fuse that activates the cancer cell.

How one responds to the invasion of the cancer cell and its rapid growth depends on the immune system and many other factors that still need to be discovered.

QUESTIONS

Q. *What evidence suggests the genetic etiology of cancer?*
A. There is clinical evidence that certain types of cancer run in families. Breast cancer is one. An inborn genetic defect (p53 gene) has recently been discovered to predispose people to breast cancer and several other cancers. The research was led by Dr. Stephen Friend of the Massachusetts General Hospital Cancer Center.

Q. *Is there other genetic evidence?*
A. Yes. Certain childhood cancers have been related to genetic defects. Wilms tumor of the kidney is one.

Q. *Does the environment play an important role in producing cancer?*
A. I believe that heredity and the environment play the most important

roles in producing cancer. I suggest that the cancer cell starts out as a mutation. (There is evidence that newborn babies come into this world with a small number of mutant cells.) As we get older, the number of mutagens increases dramatically.

Q. *What causes this dramatic increase? Is it the aging process itself? Do our organs wear out? What causes them to wear out? Is it that our immune system wears out from exposure to environmental hazards such as pesticides in our water, food and air contaminants, smoking, carbon monoxide, acid rain, increased radiation exposure, reduction of the ozone layer?*

A. I suggest that your genetic make-up will determine your destiny. Do you have oncogenes in your system or do you have the right genetic code? Do you have a strong enough immune system to combat the invasion caused by exposure to environmental hazards? In the future, we should be able to find a way to enhance immunity and conquer cancer.

Glossary of Medical Terms

Adenoma A gland-like growth, usually a benign tumor. If malignant, it is called adenocarcinoma.

Adrenal gland A small gland located just above the kidney. Its secretions (cortisone, adrenalin, aldosterone) affect the functions of other glands and organs in many important ways.

Aesthetic values. Pertaining to beauty or improvement of appearance.

Amenorrhea Absence or abnormal stoppage of the menstrual cycle (menses).

Androgen A substance, usually a hormone, that produces male characteristics (see Testosterone).

Angiogenesis The making of new blood vessels.

Anticoagulant A drug capable of slowing the clotting of blood (heparin, dicumerol, coumadin).

Aerola A pigmented ring around a central point, such as the nipple of the breast.

Aspiration A technique used to withdraw fluid or tissue through a needle from a breast tumor.

Atypical Irregular, not comforming to type. Cell that is not normal.

Autoimmune disease Disease in which the body is unable to distinguish between foreign invaders and its own tissues so it produces defensive antibodies against itself, often with serious harm.

Axillary dissection Surgical removal of lymph glands along the axillary vein and armpit.

225

Benign tumor A tumor that is not malignant (does not contain cancer).

Bilateral breast cancer Cancer involving both breasts at the same time (synchronous) or at different times (metachronous).

Biopsy Removal of a piece of tissue to be examined microscopically for diagnosis.

Bloody nipple discharge Discharge from the nipple usually detected on the underclothing and which usually indicates a benign intraductal papilloma. In rare cases it can be an indication of cancer.

Bone scan The injection of radioisotopes that concentrate in the bones and then are visualized by imaging techniques and pictures which are recorded to determine abnormalities or bone metastases (spread of breast cancer to bone).

Brachial plexus Group of interjoining nerves in the lower neck that extend to the axilla and arm.

Breast self-examination (BSE) Examination of the breasts by the woman to detect lumps visually or by palpation.

Calcification of the breast Minute calcium deposits within the breast (single or clustered) usually detected by imaging (mammography and xeromammography).

Cancer Malignant tumor. An uncontrolled growth of abnormal cells that invade and destroy the surrounding tissues.

Carcinogen A substance that can cause cancer.

Carcinoma in situ A small or minimal cancer that involves the cells on the surface and has not invaded the subcutaneous tissues.

CT Abbreviation for computerized axial tomography in which a computer is used to analyze multiple x-rays of soft body tissues.

Cathepsin D An estrogen-induced lysosomal protease. High levels may be helpful in predicting shorter metastasis-free survival and shorter disease-free survival in women with node-negative disease.

Cauterize To apply an electrical current to tissue to cut, coagulate or destroy it by heating.

CEA antigen blood test (Carcinoembryonic antigen) A nonspecific blood test used to follow breast cancer patients with metastases (spread) to determine whether the treatment method is working or not. Also used in detection and treatment of colon cancer.

Cell proliferation index Determines the rate of cells actively dividing and proliferating. Aggressive tumors have a high proportion of actively dividing (mitotic) tumors. Those tumors with a low rate have a more favorable outlook.

Chemoprevention The use of medicine or vitamins as an aid to prevent disease such as cancer.

Chemotherapy Drugs or medicine that may be used in cancer treatment that help destroy cancer cells.

Clock Palpation A method of breast self-examination using the numbers on a clock as a reference to localize lumps of any kind.

Cyst of the breast A sac filled with fluid within the breast. This can be clear yellow fluid or blood-tinged fluid and can be single or multiple.

Cytology The study of cells.

Cytotoxic Capable of being cytotoxic or poisonous to cells. Types of medicines or drugs that destroy cells.

DES (Diethylstilbestrol) A synthetic estrogen that has been used in the treatment of breast and prostate cancer. It has been associated with cancer of the vagina in the daughters of women given the compound during pregnancy and has recently been associated with an increased risk for breast cancer for mothers who took the drug.

DNA Abbreviation for deoxyribonucleic acid, a chemical in the human cell that is important in controlling heredity.

DNA Index Using a flow cytometer, the DNA content of the cell is determined. Abnormal DNA content (aneuploidy) is associated with tumors and correlates with a poor prognosis.

Doubling time The time required for a cell to duplicate itself and divide. This can apply to the breast cancer cell and has many variables depending upon the type of tumor, the host resistance, and the media in which it attempts to grow.

Duct ectasia Dilatation or widening of the ducts of the breast, often called periductal mastitis or comedomastitis. It can be associated with a nipple discharge and inflammation and can produce fibrosis and retraction of the nipple.

Dysplasia An appearance of cells that are abnormal and have features that suggest cancer but with insufficient positive changes that can be called cancer.

Edema Swelling caused by collection of fluid in tissues.

Embolus A plug or clot of blood or tumor cells within a blood vessel.

Endothelium A thin layer of cells that line the blood and lymph vessels and the chambers of the heart. Endothelial proliferation is considered necessary for tumor growth.

Epithelium Type of cells found in skin and mucous membranes.

Esophagus The tube that conveys food and liquids from the mouth to the stomach. It has a muscular lining that contracts to aid in propulsion and is lined with epithelium that secretes mucus to allow food to pass downward.

Estrogen A group of steroid female sex hormones produced primarily in the ovaries, adrenal gland, placenta, and fat tissues and essential for the development of the sexual organs and secondary sex characteristics. Synthetic estrogen is used in the birth control pills and as replacement therapy following hysterectomy and oophorectomy.

Estrogen receptor A protein that is found in target tissue cells, such as the breast, that is measured when a breast biopsy for cancer is done. The measurement of estrogen receptor is used as an aid in directing treatment of breast cancer.

Etiology Causes of disease or the study of the causes of disease.

Exogenous factors External factors that are developed and occur outside a living organism and may have a beneficial or harmful effect on that organism.

Exploratory laparotomy A surgical exploration of the abdomen to help determine the cause for life-threatening abdominal pain and discomfort (ex. appendectomy).

Fascia Thin tissues found beneath the skin between and around muscles and other structures.

Fat necrosis The destruction of fat cells usually secondary to trauma (injury) which can cause retraction of the skin or skin changes that can be confused with breast cancer.

FDA Abbreviation for Food and Drug Administration.

Fibroadenoma A fibrous firm tumor that usually occurs in young women that is almost always benign. It is usually single but can be multiple. Malignant change can develop in a fibroadenoma but is extremely rare.

Fibrocystic disease A condition seen in females usually during their menstrual years that produces fibrosis or scarring and cystic changes in the breast that are felt as lumps. These lumps appear to get larger and smaller during the menstrual cycle. The cystic changes can be single or multiple. The condition can be confused with more serious changes within the breast.

Food additives Substances that are added to food to preserve it, make it appear better, to retard deterioration, or add flavor. Some food additives are suspected carcinogens.

believed to have the ability to stop or assist in arresting the growth of the cancer cell.

Frozen section—breast A technique of freezing tissue after removing it from the breast, then cutting it into thin sections by the use of a microtone (cryostat). The tissues are then stained and mounted on a slide and looked at under the microscope to establish a diagnosis rapidly.

Galactocele Cystic enlargement of the mammary gland containing milk.

Genetic Pertaining to the origin or the beginning or the birth. Usually the term is applied to the genes that one inherits and which determine physical and mental characteristics as the organism develops.

Gynecologist A specialist in medicine who diagnoses and treats diseases of the female tract and reproductive system.

Halstead radical mastectomy The surgical removal of the breast (mastectomy) with incontinuity resection of the axillary lymph nodes and chest wall muscles (pectoralis major and minor muscles).

Hematology The medical science dealing with the study of the blood and blood diseases.

Hematoma A collection of blood that usually occurs outside a blood vessel and may be associated with a leak or injury to that vessel. The collection usually becomes clotted and may become infected. A hematoma may occur in the breast as a lump due to injury and must be watched to be sure that a more serious problem is not present.

Histology Study of the microscopic structure of cells and tissues.

Hormone A chemical substance which is secreted into the body by an endocrine gland (such as ovary or thyroid). It enters the bloodstream and plays a role in regulation of cells and tissues. (ex. estrogens, progesterone, etc.)

Host resistance The reaction of the cells or tissues of a host (immune response) to a foreign element that may threaten its existence, such as a cancer.

Hot flashes Vague sensations or vasomotor responses with the sensation of heat and sweating that is associated with the menopause.

Hypercoagulability The state of being able to clot or coagulate more easily than normal. The state of hypercoagulability may cause clumping and accumulation of elements that lead to a thrombosis or clot. Hypercoagulability may be necessary for a clumping of cancer cells to form a metastasis.

Hyperplasia A growth of cells causing an excess of cells at a specific clot. Hypercoagulability may be necessary for a clumping of cancer cells to form a metastasis.

Hyperplasia A growth of cells causing an excess of cells at a specific anatomical site (such as the ductal lining of the breast). This overgrowth may be due to hormonal stimulation, injury or chronic irritation and in the breast is seen at puberty and pregnancy. Hyperplasia is felt by some to be a premalignant change in the breast.

Hyperthyroidism An overactivity of the thyroid gland that releases excess thyroid hormones. This causes swelling of the gland, nervousness, weight loss, heat loss, tremors, and rapid heart rates.

Hypothyroidism An underactive thyroid gland that does not secrete a normal amount of thyroid hormones. This causes a deficiency state (myxedema) which produces tongue and facial swelling, dry skin, heart enlargement, voice changes, fatigue, and usually weight gain. Hypothyroidism can be caused by excessive surgical removal of the gland or disease states which affect its normal function.

Hypogammaglobulinemia Low gammaglobulins (serum protein) in the blood, which is a congenital or acquired absence of specific cells.

Hysterectomy The surgical removal of all or part of the uterus.

Immune system A complex system within the host which will resist invasion by a foreign substance (antigen) that may be harmful to the host. This is a form of protection. It is a surveillance system, and the ability of the immune system to respond can be favorable or harmful and elicits specific cellular responses.

Immunocytochemistry A chemical and cytological method using monoclonal antibodies to determine if the lymph nodes in the axilla are involved with metastatic tumor or not.

Immunosuppression A suppression of the immune system to respond. This can be normal suppression that is beneficial to the host or it can be self-destructive, producing progression of disease (ex. cancer or infection) and can be artificially induced in some cases by cytotoxic drugs or radiation.

Infiltrating ductal cancer—breast A cancer that originates in the ductal system of the breast and then breaks out of the duct and invades surrounding tissue and produces a firm fibrotic type of tumor.

Informed consent The patient being fully informed or instructed comprehensively about options in treatment in order to select the method that she wants to be used on her.

In situ breast cancer The surface cells show evidence of change indicative of cancer. There is no invasion of the subcutaneous tissue. This is a very low-grade type of breast cancer and there is no evidence of invasion or metastases.

Intraductal papilloma A benign tumor that develops within the ductal system of the breast that has papillary projections. This can cause bleeding and obstruction of the duct and can be single or multiple. It usually is benign but can be malignant.

Inversion of the nipple A turning inward or pulling inward of the nipple of the breast is usually benign or congenital but can be caused by underlying cancer.

Irradiation Treatment of disease with x-ray, radioisotope, ultraviolet, or infrared rays.

Lactation The period of time following childbirth in which the discharge of milk from the breast occurs.

Latissimus dorsi breast reconstruction flap A long muscle on the back and lateral to the breast that is used in musculocutaneous tissue transfer for reconstruction of the breast. The blood supply is kept intact. This type of reconstruction is most often used following radical mastectomy.

Liver scan A radionucleotide scan of the liver. A radioisotope is injected into a vein and concentrates in the liver and then, using a scintillation camera or rectilinear scanner, pictures are taken to detect evidence of cancer spread (metastses). Liver scan is also used as an aid in other diagnoses.

Lobular carcinoma—breast (Infiltrating or invasive.) A type of breast cancer that occurs within the terminal ducts and lobules of the breast that is invasive. It is a multicentric type of breast cancer that can be bilateral and is capable of metastases.

Lobular carcinoma in situ—breast A type of cancer that develops in premenopausal breasts in the mammary lobules and does not metastatize (spread). However, it can become invasive in a small percentage of cases.

Local excision—breast Removal of a breast lesion or tumor that is restricted to a local area within the breast. This can be done under local or general anesthesia.

Local recurrence—breast Recurrence of a breast cancer at the local site of excision or of the lumpectomy or mastectomy.

Lymph nodes Encapsulated lymph glands that are connected to the lymphatic system ducts and can be involved with breast cancer spread (metastases). (Ex. lymph glands under the armpit.)

Lymphedema of the arm A progressive swelling of the arm due to obstruction within the lymphatic system which can be crippling. Most frequently seen after radical mastectomy and radiation treatment for breast cancer.

Magnetic resonance imaging (MRI) An imaging technique that uses a magnet and electrical coil to transmit radio waves through the body to form a cross-sectional picture.

Mammography An x-ray technique to define the soft tissues of the breast. A method to produce images of the breast by low voltage x-ray to demonstrate density differences. The image is recorded on x-ray film or selenium coated plates (xeroradiography).

Mastectomy Surgical removal of all breast tissue.
a) *Simple* Removal of breast tissue only.
b) *Modified* Removal of all breast tissue and axillary lymph nodes (glands along the axillary vein and under the armpit).
c) *Patey type* Removal of all breast tissue and axillary lymph nodes and pectoralis minor muscle.
d) *Radical* Removal of all breast tissue, including chest wall muscles (pectoralis major and minor muscles) and axillary lymph nodes.

Menopause The time in the lifespan of a female when the menstrual cycle ends. Usually between the ages of 40 to 55. Ovarian function is reduced and estrogen secretion decreases or stops. A surgical menopause is due to surgical removal of the uterus and ovaries.

Metabolism The physical and chemical process by which a living organism grows, maintains its nutrition, produces energy, and its capability to reproduce.

Metastasis To form a new focus of a disease such as cancer by distant spread from its primary site. This usually occurs through lymphatic channels or blood vessels.

Micrometastases The spread of cancer that can only be seen under a microscope.

Minimal cancer Minimal cancers of the breast are nonpalpable tumors detected by mammography that measure less than 5 mm. in diameter (ex. lobular cancer in situ, intraductal cancer).

Mittelschmerz Pelvic pain that occurs in the middle of the menstrual cycle at the time of ovulation.

Monoclonal antibodies Specific antibodies derived from a single cell (cloning) which can be used to fight diseases such as cancer.

Monocyte The largest type of white blood cell, formed in the bone marrow, and capable of ingesting bacteria, viruses, and tissue debris.

Morbidity rate The number of cases per year of a specific disease per 100,000 people. Sick rate.

Morphology The study of the form and structure of an organism, organ, or its parts, including tissues and cells.

Multicentric breast cancer The development of cancer in multiple and separate areas of the breast.

Myriad An indefinite, immense number.

Necrosis The death and breakdown of tissues which are surrounded by healthy tissues.

Needle localization—breast A thin wire is introduced into the breast under x-ray control to pinpoint suspected minimal breast cancers (local anesthesia is usually used).

Neovascularization The development of blood vessels associated with tumor growth in which the lining (endothelium) of the blood vessels proliferate.

Nephrotoxic A substance such as a chemical or chemotherapeutic agent that is toxic or damaging to the structure and function of the kidneys. This damage can progress on to renal failure.

Neuroendocrine system The interaction that occurs between the nervous system and the endocrine system. An example is the hypothalamic (brain), pituitary, and adrenal gland and their effects that occur with stress.

Nuclear magnetic resonance (NMR) An imaging technique that uses a magnet and electrical coil to transmit radio waves through the body to form a cross-sectional picture.

Nucleus A spheroidal body within the cell that is separate from the cytoplasm and contains the chromosomes. It is the site of DNA replication.

Obstetrician A physician that primarily deals with the diagnosis and management of pregnancy, labor, and the postpartum care of women.

Occult cancer An obscure or hidden cancer in which the primary site can not be determined.

Omentum A fold of the lining of the abdomen containing thick, fatty fibrous tissue that extends from the stomach to adjacent organs in the abdomen (an apron type of covering over the abdominal organs).

Oncogenes Tumor genes that are present in the body that can be activated by cancer agents such as radiation or chemicals that can cause cells to become cancer.

Oncologist A physician whose specialty is the diagnosis and treatment of tumors. Most oncologists have had additional specialized training in a major cancer center.

Oophorectomy The surgical removal of an ovary or ovaries.

Osteoporosis A condition that most commonly affects women after the menopause in which there is a washing out or demineralization of bone that can cause pain and deformity of the spine. Pathological fractures (breaks) can develop.

Ovaries Two female reproductive glands, containing the ova or germ cells.

Paget's Disease of the nipple A ductal cancer of the breast that involves the skin of the nipple and areola. A crusty, scaly, red dermatitis type of lesion.

Palpation Examination by feeling with the hand.

Parenchyma Specific tissue of an animal organ as distinguished from its connective or supporting tissue.

Pathology The branch of medicine which deals with the changes in the body produced by disease.

Pectoralis muscles Pectoralis major and minor muscles directly under the breast and attached to the chest wall. The muscles removed in a radical mastectomy.

Pelvic inflammatory disease (PID) An acute or chronic inflammatory disease of the pelvic organs which occurs predominately in young sexually active females and can lead to infertility.

Percentage of cells in S-phase Indicates the number of cells in a tumor actively making DNA. If there is a high fraction of S-phase cells in a tumor showing poor differentiation, the tumor may have a poorer prognosis.

Pesticides Poisons used to destroy pests that inhibit the growth of plants or animals (ex. insecticides, fungicides, rodenticides).

Pleomorphism The unusual, irregular, and abnormal cell and nuclear shapes that occur in various distinct forms of the cancer cells.

Pleural effusion The collection of fluid between the serous membrane that covers the lungs (visceral pleura) and the lining of the chest (parental pleura) cavity (thorax).

Progesterone A female sex hormone secreted by the ovaries that prepares the uterus for pregnancy and the breasts for lactation.
Progestin is the synthetic form of progesterone.

Progestogen is a substance prossessing progestational actively and is also used in oral contraceptives.

Prolactin A hormone in the pituitary gland that stimulates lactation and the production of progesterone by the ovaries. Measured by radio-immune assay technique.

Prophylactic castration The removal of the ovaries in patients with breast cancer to, hopefully, prevent metastases. Also used in the treatment of breast cancer after spread has occurred.

Prophylactic subcutaneous mastectomy Removing all of the breast tissue subcutaneously as a preventive measure for breast cancer. This is a misnomer, since it is almost impossible to remove all breast tissue with this operation.

Prosthetic device A device that serves as a substitute, such as a silicone gel plastic bag, to replace the mound of the breast after mastectomy.

Quadrectomy Excision of approximately one-fourth of the breast tissue.

Radiation A stream of particles emitted by a radioactive material. This can be used for diagnostic purposes of treatment and the biological effects can be both helpful and harmful.

Radioisotope An isotope that is radioactive. Injection of isotopes which concentrate in the bones or liver are used to detect spread of breast cancer (metastases to that site).

Red blood cells Red blood cells are formed in the bone marrow. Their main function is oxygen transport and they survive for approximately 120 days in the circulation.

Regional metastases Spread of a primary cancer to a regional site, such as breast cancer spreading to the lymph nodes under the armpit.

Rehabilitation Restoring a person to healthy, useful activity following surgery such as mastectomy.

Replacement hormone therapy The use of hormones such as estrogen to replace the natural hormones lost when an oophorectomy (ovaries) and hysterectomy (uterus) is done.

Scintillation camera Device used to magnify radiation and record the results for the diagnosis of cancer or other disorders.

Scirrhous cancer—breast A cancer of the breast with a hard, firm, fibrous consistency, usually an infiltrating ductal carcinoma, that can be confused with other diagnoses.

Screening mammography A female over a specified age (40 years) has a mammography done as a routine procedure, usually once a year, to see if the breast is involved with cancer.

Silicone Synthetic compound used in breast implants because of its flexibility, resilience, and tensile strength. Usually a gel inside a plastic bag.

Skin dimpling The indentation of the skin, which can be seen, that indicates the possibility of a cancer in the breast. Usually due to ligaments just under the skin surface that are involved with cancer and are attached to the skin.

Slough A mass or layer of dead tissue which separates from the surrounding or underlying living tissue.

Stage of breast disease A method of staging breast cancer based on the size of the tumor, whether regional axillary lumph nodes are involved, whether skin, chest muscles, distant lymph nodes or bloodstream spread has occurred.

Systemic disease As related to breast disease, means that the primary tumor has disseminated and spread to distal sites, such as the liver, chest, brain, bones, or soft tissues.

Tamoxifen An estrogen blocking agent (drug) used in the preventive and prophylastic treatment of breast cancer.

Thermography A method of measuring temperature variations in the breast that may contain cancer. Breast tumors show up as "hot spots" on the thermogram.

Thrombin An enzyme which is necessary for blood to clot.

Thrombophlebitis A clot that usually forms in a vein and causes an inflammatory response. The clot is usually due to stasis or pooling of blood and occurs most often in the lower extremities and pelvis.

Thyroid gland Gland located in the lower neck that plays a large role in metabolic functions. The gland can become enlarged due to stress or hyper- or hypo-functioning. Normal iodine intake is necessary for normal function.

Triglycerides Form in which dietary fat is stored in the body, consisting of glycerol combined with three fatty-acid molecules.

Tummy tuck—breast reconstruction Resection of the lower skin of the abdomen with the blood supply (rectus muscles) transplanted to the chest wall and breast area and used for breast reconstruction and abdominal cosmesis.

Ultrasonography (ultrasound) A method in which high-frequency sound waves are used to outline anatomical structures of the body. High-frequency sounds are transmitted through the body and the echoes are detected and displayed on a television screen. It is used primarily to determine if a structure is solid or liquid and is useful in detecting breast cysts in young females with firm fibrous breasts (no radiation effect occurs).

Uterus The womb or hollow muscular organ lined by epithelium in the pelvis that receives and holds the fertilized egg. It feeds and nourishes the developing embryo and fetus. Removed during hysterectomy.

Vaginitis—atrophic An inflammation of the vagina that occurs after menopause in which the vaginal tissue becomes thin and dry due to decreased estrogen production.

White blood cells The cells in the blood that remain after the red cells have been removed. The white cells play a role in defense against infection and T-cell lymphocytes and B-cell lymphocytes (a part of the total number of white cells) play a role in the immune system against cancer.

Xeroradiography X-ray imaging technique in which images of breast tissue are reproduced on a xerox plate rather than on conventional x-ray film.

Sources for Further Information

American Cancer Society
4 West 35th Street
New York, NY 10001
Phone: 800–ACS–2345

American Medical Association
515 N. State St.
Chicago, IL 60610

Breast Cancer Support and
  Information Hot Line
Y-ME
Phone: 800–221–2141 or 312–
  799–8228

Cancer Information Service
National Cancer Institute
Bethesda, MD 20205
Phone: 800–422–6237 or 800–
  638–6694

Consumer Information Center
U.S. Government Printing
  Office
Pueblo, CO 81009

Memorial Sloan-Kettering
  Cancer Center
Early Detection Phone Line
Phone: 800–DETECT5

National Alliance of Breast
  Cancer Organizations
  (NABCO)
1180 Avenue of the Americas,
  2nd Floor
New York, NY 10036

Comprehensive Cancer Centers

University of Alabama in
  Birmingham
Comprehensive Cancer Center

University of Southern
California
Comprehensive Cancer Center
1441 Eastlake Avenue
Los Angeles, CA 90033
Phone: 213–224–6416

Fox Chase Cancer Center
University of Pennsylvania
7701 Burholme Avenue
Philadelphia, PA 19111

Columbia University Cancer
Research Center
701 W. 168th Street
New York, NY 10032
Phone: 212–694–3647

Comprehensive Cancer Center
for the State of Florida
University of Miami School of
Medicine
1475 N.W. 12th Avenue
Miami, FL 33101
Phone: 305–545–7707

Dana-Farber Cancer Institute
44 Binney Street
Boston, MA 02115
Phone: 617–732–3555

Duke Comprehensive Cancer
Center
P.O. Box 3814
Duke University Medical Center
Durham, NC 27710
Phone: 919–684–2282

Georgetown University
Comprehensive Breast Center
Lombardi Building
3800 Reservoir Road N.W.
Washington, DC 20007
Phone: 202-687-2104

Johns Hopkins Oncology Center
600 North Wolfe Street
Baltimore, MD 21205
Phone: 301–955–8822

Fred Hutchinson Cancer
Research Center
1124 Columbia Street
Seattle, WA 98104
Phone: 206–292–2930

Illinois Cancer Council
36 S. Wabash Avenue
Chicago, IL 60603
Phone: 312–346–9813

Mayo Clinic
200 First Street S.W.
Rochester, MN 55905
Phone: 507–284–8964

Memorial Sloan-Kettering
Cancer Center
1275 York Avenue
New York, NY 10021
Phone: 212–794–6561

Michigan Cancer Foundation
Meyer L. Prentis Cancer Center
110 East Warren Avenue
Detroit, MI 48201
Phone: 313–833–0710

Ohio State University
Comprehensive Cancer
Center
410 West 12th Avenue
Columbus, OH 43210
Phone: 614–422–5022

Roswell Park Memorial Institute
666 Elm Street
Buffalo, NY 14263
Phone: 716–845–5770

The University of Texas System
  Cancer Center
M.D. Anderson Hospital and
  Tumor Institute
6723 Bertner Avenue
Houston, TX 77030
Phone: 713-792-6000

UCLA-Jonsson Comprehensive
  Cancer Center
Louis Factor Health Sciences
  Bldg.
10833 LeConte Ave.
Los Angeles, CA 90024
Phone: 213-825-5268

Lurleen Wallace Tumor Institute
1824 6th Ave. S.
Birmingham, AL 35294
Phone: 205-934-5077

Wisconsin Clinical Cancer
  Center
University of Wisconsin
600 Highland Avenue
Madison, WI 53792
Phone: 608-263-8610

Yale Comprehensive Cancer
  Center
Yale University School of
  Medicine
New Haven, CT 06510
Phone: 203-785-4095

Drugs and Radiation

Food and Drug Administration
5600 Fishers Lane
Rockville, MD 20857
Phone: 202-872-0382

Medisense
1133 Avenue of the Americas
New York, NY 10036

Public and Professional Affairs
U.S. Pharmacopeia
12601 Twinbrook Parkway
Rockville, MD 20852

Food and Nutrition

American Council on Science
  and Health
47 Maple Street
Summit, NJ 07901

American Institute for Cancer
  Research
Washington, DC 20069

American Institute of Nutrition
9650 Rockville Pike
Bethesda, MD 20014

Center for Science in the Public
  Interest
1755 S. Street N.W.
Washington, DC 20009

Consumer Food Safety
Department of Agriculture
Washington, DC 20250
Phone: 202-472-4485

Food Safety Council
1725 K Street, N.W.
Washington, DC 20006

Gynecology and Obstetrics

American College of
  Obstetricians and
  Gynecologists
600 Maryland Avenue, S.W.
Washington, DC 20024
Phone: 202-638-5577

Center for Reproductive and
Sexual Health
424 East 62nd Street
New York, NY 10021

National Women's Health
Network
224 Seventh Street, S.E.
Washington, DC 20003
Phone: 202–543–9222

Planetree Health Resource
Center
2040 Webster Street
San Francisco, CA 94115
Phone: 415–346–4636

Public Health

American Public Health
Association
1015 15th Street, N.W.
Washington, DC 20005

Center for Medical Consumers
237 Thompson Street
New York, NY 10012
Phone: 212–674–7105

Consumer Health Information
Center
680 East 600 South
Salt Lake City, UT 84103
Phone: 801–364–9318

National Health Information
Clearinghouse
U.S. Public Health Service
Washington, DC 20013
Phone: 800–336–4797

Personal Health Record
Metropolitan Life Insurance
Company
One Madison Avenue
New York, NY 10010

President's Council on Physical
Fitness
450 5th Street, N.W.
Washington, DC 20036
Phone: 202–872–0382

Public Citizen Health Research
Group
200 P Street, N.W.
Washington, DC 20036
Phone: 202–872–0382

World Health Organization
Room 2427
United Nations, NY 10017

Rehabilitation and Counseling

American Family Therapy
Association
15 Bond Street
Great Neck, NY 11021

Breast Cancer Advisory Center
Box 224
Kensington, MD 20795

Cancer Counseling and Research
1300 Summit Avenue
Fort Worth, TX 76102
Phone: 817–335–4823

Family Service Association of
America
44 East 23rd Street
New York, NY 10010

Mental Health Clearinghouse
5600 Fishers Lane
Rockville, MD 20857
Phone: 202–443–4513

National Genetic Foundation
55 West 57th Street
New York, NY 10019

National Self-Help
  Clearinghouse
33 West 42nd Street
New York, NY 10036
Phone: 212–840–7606

Reach to Recovery
American Cancer Society
4 West 34th Street
New York, NY 10001
Phone: 212–736–3030

Surgery and Reconstruction

American College of Surgeons
55 East Erie Street
Chicago, IL 60611

American Society of Plastic and
  Reconstructive Surgeons
233 North Michigan Avenue
Chicago, IL 60601
Phone: 800–635–0635

American Surgical Association
32 Fruit Street
Boston, MA 02114

Association of American
  Physicians and Surgeons
8991 Cotswold Drive
Burke, VA 22015

Coalition for the Medical Rights
  of Women
1638 Haight Street
San Francisco, CA 94117

Miscellaneous

Encore Program
YWCA
726 Broadway
New York, NY 10003

National Center for Health
  Statistics
3700 East-West Highway
Hyattsville, MD 20782
Phone: 301–436–7085

National Institutes of Health
9000 Rockville Pike
Bethesda, MD 20892

Health and Human Services
  Department
3700 East-West Highway
Hyattsville, MD 20782
Phone: 301–436–6716

References

1. Wilson, R. E.; Donegan, W. L.; Mettlin, C.; Nachimuthu, N.; Stuart, C. R.; Murphy, G. P., "The 1982 National Survey of the Breast in the United States by the American College of Surgeons." *Surg. Gyn., Obst.* (October 1984) Vol. 159, 4, p. 309–317.
2. Axtell, L. M.; Asire, A. J.; Myers (eds), Cancer patient survival. Rep. No. 5 *DHEW* Pub. No. (NIH) 77–992. Besthesda, National Cancer Institute, 1976.
3. Merkel, Douglas E., Osborne, C. Kent, Issues in the Management of Breast Cancer, *Advances in Oncol.* 1987, Vol. 4, No. 3, p. 9–16.
4. Silverberg, E.; Lubera, J. A., Cancer Statistics, 1988, Ca, 1988: 38:5–22.
5. Sigurdsson, Helgi, et al. Indicators of Prognosis in Node-Negative Breast Cancer, *New Eng. J. Med.*, April 12, 1990, Vol. 322, No. 15, p. 1045–1053.
6. Diet and Health, National Academy Press, Wash., D.C. 1989, p. 206–208.
7. Diet and Health, Nat'l Ac. Press, Wash., D.C. 1989, p. 579–580.
8. Rouviere, H., Anatomie des Lymphatiques de L'homme Paris, Masson, et cie, 1932, p. 197–240.
9. Rotter, J., Zur Topographie des mamma-carcinomas. *Arch. Klin. Chir.*, 1899, 58:346.
10. Sappey, P. C., *Anatomie, Physiolgie, Patholgoie des Vaisseauz Lymphatique Consideres chez l' Homme et les Vertbris.* Paris: A. Delahaye and E. Lecrosnie 18, [74] 85.
11. Lilienfeld, Abraham M., The epidemiology of breast cancer. *Cancer Res.* 1963, 23:1503.
12. Macklin, Madge T. Comparison of the number of breast cancer deaths observed in relatives of breast cancer patients, and the number expected on the basis of mortality rates. *J. Nat'l. Cancer Inst.*, 1959, 22:927.
13. Fraumeni, J. F., Jr., Lloyd, J. W.; Smith, E. M.; and Wagoner, J. K., Cancer mortality among nuns: Role of marital status in etiology of neoplastic disease in women. *J. Nat'l Cancer Inst.* 1969, 42:455.

14. Trichopoulos, D.; MacMahon, B.; and Cole, P., Menopause and breast cancer risk. *J. Nat'l Cancer Inst.* 1972, 48:605.

15. International Agency for Research on Cancer. Sex hormones (11). IARC Monogr. Eval. Carcinog. *Risk Chem Hum*, 1979; 21:5–583.

16. Bergkvist, Leif, et al, The Risk of Breast Cancer after Estrogen and Estrogen-Progestin Replacement, *New Eng. J. Med.*, Aug 3, 1989, Vol. 321, No. 5, p. 293–297.

17. Persson I.; Adami H-O.; Bergkvist L. et al., Risk of endometrial cancer after treatment with estrogens alone or in conjunction with progestogens: results of a prospective study. *Br. Med. J.* 1989; 298:147–51.

18. Finley, J. W. and Bogardus, G. M., Breast cancer and thyroid disease. *Quart. Rev. Surg.* 1960, 17:139–147.

19. Stadel, B. V., Dietary iodine and risk of breast, endometrial, and ovarian cancer. *Lancet* 1976, 1:890–891.

20. Backwinkel, L. and Jackson, A. S., Some features of breast cancer and thyroid deficiency—report of 280 cases. *Cancer.* 1964, 17:1174–1176.

21. Graham, S.; Levin, M.; and Lilienfeld, A., The socio-economic distribution of cancer in various sites in Buffalo, NY, 1948–1952. *Cancer.* 1960, 13:180–191.

22. Gallup, Omnibus., A survey concerning cigarette smoking, health check-ups, cancer: The American Cancer Society Inc., The Gallup Organization Inc., GO 7695 T. January, 1977.

23. Egan, Robert L., *Breast Imaging: Diagnosis and Morphology of Breast Diseases* 1988, W.B. Saunders p. 531.

24. Kurt J. M., et al, France *Int. J. Radiat. Oncol., Biol., Phys.* 1988, 15:277–84.

25. Humphrey, Loren J., Multidisciplinary cancer care. *Oncology Times*, May, 1983, Vol. V, No. 5.

26. Martin, Hayes E., and Ellis, Edward B., Biopsy by needle puncture and aspiration. 1930, *Ann. Surg.* 32:169.

27. Saphir, Otto., Early diagnosis of breast lesions. *J.A.M.A.*, 1952, Vol. 150, No. 9, 859–861.

28. Robbins, G. F.; Brothers, J. H., III; Eberhart, W. F.; and Quan, S., Is aspiration biopsy of the breast cancer dangerous to patients? *Cancer*, 1974, 7:774–778.

29. Berg, John W., and Robbins, G. F., A late look at the safety of aspiration biopsy. *Cancer*, 1962, 15:826–7.

30. Vorherr, H., Study indicates that multihole needle may be more accurate for breast aspiration biopsy. *Oncology Times*, Dec. 1983, Vol. V, No. 12, p. 4.

31. Kreuzer, G. and Zajicek, J., Cytologic diagnosis of mammary tumors from aspiration biopsy smears 111 studies on 200 carcinomas with false negative or doubtful cytologic reports. *Acta Cytol* 1972, 16:249.

32. Drexler, B.; Davis, J. L.; Schofield, G., Diaphanography in the diagnosis of breast cancer. *Radiology* 1985, 157:41.

33. Ries, E. (1930): Diagnostic lipoidal injection into milk ducts followed by infection. *Am. J. Obstet. Gynecol.*, 20:414.

34. Gautherie, Michel and Gross, Charles M., Breast thermography and cancer risk prediction. *Cancer*, 1980. 45:51–56.

35. Stark, A. M. and Way, S., The screening of well women for the early detection of breast cancer using clinical examinations with thermography and mammography. *Cancer*, 1974, 33:1671–1679.

36. Wallace, J. D. and Dodd, G. D., Thermography in the diagnosis of breast cancer. *Radiology*, 1968, 91:679–685.
37. Wild, J. J. and Neal D., The use of high frequency ultrasonic waves for detecting changes of texture in living tissue. *Lancet*, 1951, 1:655.
38. Wild, J. J. and Reid, J. M., Further pilot echographic studies on the histologic structure of the living intact breast. *Am. J. Pathol.*, 1952, 28:839.
39. Kobayashi, T., Review: Ultrasonic diagnosis of breast cancer. *Ultrasound Med. Biol.*, 1975, 1:383.
40. Ruzicka, Francis F., Jr.; Kaufman, Leonard; Shapiro, Gerald; Perez, Joseph V.; and Grossi, Carlo, E., Xeromammography and film mammography—A comparative study. *Radiology*, 1965, 85:260–269.
41. Wolfe, John N., Xerography of the breast. *Radiology*, 1968. 91:231–240.
42. Martin, John E. and Gallagher, H. Stephen, Mammographic diagnosis of minimal breast cancer. *Cancer*, 1971, 28:1519–1526.
43. Frankl, Gloria and Rosenfeld, David D., Xeroradiographic detection of occult breast cancer. *Cancer*, 1975, 35:542–548.
44. Salomon, A., Beitrage zur Pathologies und Klinik des Mammakarzinoms. *Arch. Klin. Chir.*, 1913, 101:573.
45. Warren, S. L., A roentgenologic study of the breast. *Am. J. Roentgenol*, 1950, 24:113.
46. Egan, R. L., Experience with mammography in a tumor institution. *Radiology*, 1960, 74:894.
47. Clark, R. L., Copeland, M. M.; Egan, R. L. et al., Reproductibility of the technic of mammography (Egan) for cancer of the breast. *Am. J. Surg.*, 1965, 109:127.
48. Black, F., Physical Review, 1946, 70:460–474.
49. Purcell, E M.; Torrey, H. C.; Pound, R. V., *Physical Reviews*, 1946, 69:37–38.
50. Doyle, F. H.; Gore, J. C.; Perrnock, J. M. et al 1981, *Lancet* 53, 57.
51. Wells, C. A.; Heryet, A.; Brochier, J.; Gatter, K. C.; and Mason, D. Y., The immunocytochemical detection of axillary micrometastases in breast cancer. *Br. J. Cancer*, 1984, 50:193–197.
52. Friedman, Nathan B., Pathologist warns radiation therapy not conservative, hits healthy tissue. *Hospital Tribune Report*, July 18, 1984, p. 18.
53. Mettler, Fred A., Jr.; Hempelmann, Louis H.; Dutton, Arthur M.; Pifer, James, W.; Toyooka, Edward T.; Ames, Wendell R., Breast neoplasms in women treated with x-rays for acute postpartum mastitis. A pilot study. *J. Nat'l. Cancer Inst.*, 1969, 43:803–811.
54. Dvoretsky, Philip M.; Woodard, Elizabeth; Bonfiglio, Thomas A.; Hempelmann, Louis H.; and Morse, Ilka P., The pathology of breast cancer in women irradiated for acute postpartum mastitis. *Cancer*, 1980, 46:2257–2262.
55. Mackenzie, I., Breast cancer following multiple fluoroscopies. *Br. J. Ca.*, 1965, 19:1–8.
56. Wanebo, C. K.; Johnson, K. G.; Sato, K.; and Thorslund, T. W., Breast cancer after exposure to the atomic bombings of Hiroshima and Nagasaki. *New Eng. J. Med.*, 1968, Vol. 279, No. 13, 667–671.
57. Hildreth, Nancy, G., et al., The risk of breast cancer after irradiation of the thymus in infancy. *New Eng. J. Med.*, Nov. 9, 1989, Vol. 321, No. 19, 1281–1290.
58. Beir Report. Advisory Committee on the Biological Effects of ionizing radiations. National Academy of Sciences—National Research Council: The effects on popula-

tions of exposure to low levels of ionizing radiation. U.S. Gov't Print. Off., Washington, D.C., 1972.

59. Kopans, Daniel B., Fine-needle aspiration of clinically occult breast lesions. *Radiology* 1989; 170:313–314.

60. Urrutia, Enrique J., et al., Retractable—Barb needle for breast lesion localization: Use in 60 cases. *Radiology* 1988; 169:845–847.

61. Horns, J. W.; Arndt, R. D., Percutaneous spot localization of nonpalpable breast lesions. *A.S.R.* 1976; 127:253–256.

62. Gent, H. J., et al., Stereotaxic needle localization and cytological diagnosis of occult breast lesions. *Ann. Surg.* Nov. 1986, Vol. 204, No. 5, p. 580–584.

63. Hutchinson, W. B.; Thomas, D. B.; Hamlin, W. B.; Roth, G. J.; Peterson, A. V.; Williams, B., Risk of breast cancer in women with benign breast disease. *J.N.C.I.* July 1980, Vol. 65, No. 1, 13–20.

64. Soini, I.; Aine, R.; Lauslahti, K.; Hakama, M., Independent risk factors of benign and malignant breast lesions. *Amer. J. Epidemiology*, 1981, Vol. 114, No. 4, 507–512.

65. Haas, Ann F. and Bodai, Balazs I., Carcinoma of the breast arising in a fibroadenoma: Report of three cases and a review of the literature. *Contemporary Surgery*, Vol. 36, March 1990, p. 63–65.

66. Fondo, E. Y.; Rosen, P. P.; Fracchia, A. A.; Urban, J. A., The problem of carcinoma developing in a fibroadenoma: Recent experience at Memorial Hospital. *Cancer*, 1979, 43:563–567.

67. Buzanowski-Konakry, K.; Harrison, E. G., Jr.; Payne, W. S., Lobular carcinoma arising in fibroadenoma of the breast. *Cancer*, 1975, 35:450–456.

68. Kodijin, D.; Winger, E. E.; Morgenstern, N. L.; Chen. U., Chronic mastopathy and breast cancer. A follow-up study. *Cancer*, 1977, 39:2603–2607.

69. Riberio, C. G. and Palmer, M. K., Breast carcinoma associated with pregnancy: A clinician's dilemma. *Br. Med. J.*, 1977, 2:1524–27.

70. Donegan, W. L., Breast cancer and pregnancy. *Obstet. Gynecol*, 1977, 50:244–252.

71. Donegan, W. L., Cancer and pregnancy. *Ca.—A cancer journal for clinicians*, 1983, 33:195–214.

72. Gent, H. J.; Sprenger, E.; Dowlatshahi, K., Stereotaxic Needle Localization and Cytological Diagnosis of Occult Breast Lesions. *Ann. Surg.* Nov. 1986, Vol. 204, No. 5, p. 580–584.

73. Barber, H. R. K. and Braber, E. A., *Surgical disease in pregnancy*. Philadelphia, W. B. Saunders Company, 1974, 303–309, 728–729.

74. Dilman, V. M., Metabolic immunodepression which increases the risk of cancer. *Lancet*, Dec. 10, 1977, 1207–1209.

75. White, T. T., Carcinoma of the breast in the pregnant and the nursing patient. Review of 1375 cases. *Am. J. Obstet, Gynec.* 1955, 69:1277–1286.

76. Jones, R. and Wernerman, B., MOPP (nitrogen mustard, vincristine, procarbazine and prednisone) given during pregnancy. *Obstet. Gynecol.* 1979, 54:477–478.

77. Geggie, Peter, H. S., Breast cancer in pregnant women. *C.M.A. Journal*, Sept. 1, 1982, 127:358–359.

78. MacMahon, B.; Lin, T. M.; Lowe, C. R., et al., Lactation and cancer of the breast, a summary of an international study. *Bull. W.H.O.* 1970, 42:185–194.

79. Lee, T. N. and Horz, J. M., Significance of ovarian metastases in therapeutic oophorectomy for advanced breast cancer. *Cancer*, 1971, 27:1374–1378.

80. Kennedy, B. J.; Mielke, P. W.; Fortuny, I. E., Therapeutic abortion versus prophylactic castration in mammary carcinoma. *Surg. Gynec. Obstet.*, 1964, 118:524–540.

81. Greenberg, E. R.; Barnes, A. B.; Resseguie, L.; Barrett, J. A.; Burnside, S.; Lanza, L. L.; Neff, R. K.; Stevens, M.; Young, R. H.; Colton, T., Breast cancer in mothers given Diethylstilbestrol in pregnancy. *New Eng. J. Med.* 1984, 311–1393–8.

82. White, T. T., Prognosis of breast cancer for pregnant and nursing women: analysis of 1413 cases. *Surg. Gynecol. Obstet.*, 1955, 100:661.

83. Rissanen, P. M., Carcinoma of the breast during pregnancy and lactation. *Br. J. Cancer*, 1968, 22:663.

84. Peters, M. V., The effect of pregnancy in breast cancer in: Prognostic factors in breast cancer. Edited by A. P. M. Forest and P. B. Kunkler, London: E. & S. Livingstone 1968, p. 65–80.

85. Harvey, J. C.; Rosen, P. P.; Ashikari, R.; Robbins, G. F.; Kinne, D. W., The effect of pregnancy on the prognosis of carcinoma of the breast following radical mastectomy. *Surg. Gynecol. Obstet.*, 1981, 153:723–725.

86. Osbourne, C. Kent, DNA Flow Cytometry in Early Breast Cancer: A step in the right direction. *Journal of the National Cancer Institute*, 1989, Vol. 81, No. 18, p. 1344–5.

87. Abeloff, Martin D.; Beveridge, Ray A., Adjuvant Chemotherapy of breast cancer—the consensus development conference revisited. *Oncology*, 1988, Vol. 2, No. 4, p. 21–26.

88. Weidfner, N.; Semple, S. P.; Welch, W. R.; Folkman, J., Tumor Angiogenesis and Metastasis—Correlation in Invasive Breast Carcinoma. *New Eng. J. Med.*, 1991, 324:1–8.

89. Halsted, W. S., The treatment of wounds with special reference to the value of the blood clot in the management of dead spaces. *Johns Hopkins Hospital Reports*, 1891, 2:255–316.

90. Roentgen, W. C., On a new kind of rays. *Clinical Orthopedics and related research* (New York: J. B. Lippincott Co.) 1969, 65:3–8.

91. Kraft, E. and Finby, N., Wilhelm Conrad Roentgen (1845–1923) Discoverer of x-ray. 1974, 74:2066–70.

92. McWhirter, R., Simple mastectomy and radiotherapy in the treatment of breast cancer. *Brit. J. Radiol.* March 1955, 28:128–139.

93. Stewart, H. J. and Sutherland, I., *World J. Surg.* 1976.

94. Stewart, H. J., Controlled trials in the treatment of "early" breast cancer: A review of published results. *World J. Surg.* 1977, 1:309–313.

95. Bonadonna, G.; Brusamolino, E.; Valagussa, P.; Rossi, A.; Brugnatelli, L.; Brambilla, C.; DeLena, M.; Tancini, G.; Bajetta, E.; Musumeci, R.; Veronesi, U., Combination chemotherapy as an adjuvant treatment in operable breast cancer. *N. Eng. J. Med.* 1976, 294:405–410.

96. Peters, M. V., Wedge resection and irradiation—an effective treatment in early breast cancer. *J.A.M.A.*, 1967, 200:144–145.

97. Meyer, K. K.; Weaver, D. R.; Luft, W. C.; Boselli, B. D., Lymphocyte immune deficiency following irradiation for carcinoma of the breast. *Front. Radiation Ther. Onc.* 1972, 7, 179, edit. J. M. Vaeth; S. Karger; Basel.

98. Slater, J. M.; Ngo, E.; and Lau, B. H. S., Effect of therapeutic irradiation on the immune responses. *Amer. J. Roentgenol*, 1976, 126, 313.

99. Effects of Adjuvant Tamoxifen and of Cytotoxic Therapy on Mortality in Early Breast Cancer. *N. Eng. J. Med.* 1988; 319:1681–92.

100. Rosenberg, S. A.; Lotze, M. T.; Muul, L. M. et al., Observations on the systemic administration of autologous lymphokine activated killer cells and recombinant interleukin-2 to patients with metasatic cancer. *N. Eng. J. Med.*, 1985, 313:1485.

101. Rosenblum, M. G.; Lamki, L. M.; Murray, J. L.; Carlo, D. G.; Gutterman, J. U., Interferon—induced changes in pharmacokinetic and tumor uptake of 111 In-labeled antimelanoma antibody 96.5 in melanoma patients. *J. Natl Cancer Inst.* 1988, 80:160–165.

102. Swain, S. M., Ductal Carcinoma in situ—Incidence, Presentation, Guidelines to Treatment. *Oncology* March 1989 Vol. 3, No. 3., p. 29.

103. Fisher, E. R.; Sass, R.; Fisher, B. et al., Pathologic findings from the National Surgical Adjuvant Breast Project Protocol 6. Intraductal Carcinoma (DCIS) *Cancer*, 1986, 57:197–208.

104. Rosner, D.; Bedwani, R. N.; Vana, J. et al., Noninvasive breast carcinoma: Results of a National Survey by the American College of Surgeons. *Ann. Surg.*, 1980, 192:139–147.

105. Swain, S. M. and Lippmann, M. E., Intraepithelial Carcinoma of the Breast: Molecular Carcinoma in situ and Ductal Carcinoma in situ. In: Lippman, M. E.; Lichter, A. S.; Danforth, D. N., (eds), *The Diagnosis and Management of Breast Cancer*, 1988, p. 296–325. Philadelphia: WB Saunders Co.

106. Frykberg, E. R.; Santiago, F.; Betsil, W. L.; O'Brien, P. H., Lobular carcinoma in situ of the breast. *Surg. Gynecol. Obstet.*, 1987, 164:285–301.

107. Haagensen, C. D.; Lane, N.; Lattes, R.; Bodian, C., Lobular neoplasia (so-called lobular carcinoma in situ) of the breast. *Cancer*, 1978, 42:737–769.

108. Swain, S. M.; Lippmann, M. E., Intraepithelial carcinoma of the breast: Molecular Carcinoma in situ and Ductal Carcinoma in situ. In: Lippmann, M.E.; Lichter, A. S.; Danforth, D. N. (eds): *The Diagnosis and Management of Breast Cancer* 1988, p. 296–325, Philadelphia: W. B. Saunders Co.

109. Farrow, J. H., The James Ewing lecture: Current Concepts in the Detection and Treatment of the earliest of the early breast cancers. *Cancer*, 1970, 25:468–477.

110. Newman, W., In situ lobular carcinoma of the breast: Report of 26 women with 32 cancers. *Ann. Surg.*, 1963, 157:591–599.

111. Urban, J. A., Biopsy of the "normal" breast in treating breast cancer. *Surg. Clin. N. Amer.*, 1969, 49:291–301.

112. Rosen, P. P.; Senil, R.; Schottenfeld, D.; Ashikari, R., Noninvasive breast carcinoma: Frequency of unsuspected invasion and implications for treatment. *Ann. Surg.* 1979, 189:377–382.

113. Giordano, J. M. and Klopp, C. T., Lobular carcinoma in situ: Incidence and treatment. *Cancer* 1973, 31:105–109.

114. Silverstein, M. J.; Warsiman, J. R.; Greison, E. D.; Colburn, W. J.; Gamagami, P.; Lewinsky, B. S., Radiation Therapy for Intraductal Carcinoma—Is it an Equal Alternative? Presented at the Forty-Third Annual Cancer Symposium, The Society of Surgical Oncology, Washington, D.C. May 20, 1990.

115. Fisher, B.; Bauer, M.; Margolese, R.; Poisson, R.; Pilch, Y.; Redmond, C.; Fisher, E.; Wolmark, N.; Deutsch, M.; Montague, E.; Saffer, E.; Wickerham, L.; Lernes, H.; Glass, A.; Shibata, H.; Deckers, P.; Ketcham, A.; Oishi, R.; Russell, I., Five-

year results of a randomized clinical trial comparing total mastectomy and segmental mastectomy with or without radiation in the treatment of breast cancer. *New Eng. J. Med.*, March 14, 1985, 312:665–673.

116. Davis, J. B., Carcinoma of the breast. Arch. Surg. 1957, 74:758–769.
117. Farrow, J. H.; Fracchia, A. A.; Robbins, G. F.; Castro, E., Simple excision or biopsy plus radiation therapy as the primary treatment for potentially curable cancer of the breast. *Cancer*, 1971, 28:1195–1201.
118. Pigott, J.; Nichols, R.; Maddox, W. A.; Balch, C. M. (Univ. of Alabama Med. Center, Birmingham) *Surg. Gynecol. Obstet.* March 1984, 158:255–259.
119. Gallagher, H. S. and Martin, J. E., Early phases in the development of breast cancer. *Cancer*, 1969, 24:1170–1178.
120. Rosen, P. P.; Fracchia, A. A.; Urban, J. A.; Schottenfeld, D.; Robbins, G. F., Residual mammary carcinoma following simulated partial mastectomy. *Cancer* 1975, 35:739–47.
121. Lesser, M. L.; Rosen, P. P.; Kinne, D. W., Multicentricity and bilaterality in invasive breast carcinoma. *Surgery* 1982, 91:234–240.
122. Peters, M. V., Wedge resection and irradiation—an effective treatment in early breast cancer. *J.A.M.A.*, 1967, 200:144–145.
123. Conservation Equal to Mastectomy in treatment of Early Breast Cancer. *Oncology and Biotechnology News*, August 1990.
124. Sesto, Mark E., et al., Early Hospital Discharge Following Mastectomy: 239 Consecutive Patients Over Three Years. *Contemporary Surgery*, Sept. 1989 35:37–40.
125. The Ludwig Breast Cancer Study Group. Prolonged disease free survival after one course of perioperative adjuvant chemotherapy for node-negative breast cancer. *New Eng. J. Med.*, 1989; 320:491–6.
126. Sternberg, Steve, Breast Cancer Treatments Disputed. *Atlanta Constitution*, Tues. Oct. 17, 1989.
127. Hermann, Robert E., et al, Cleveland Clinic Foundation. The Changing Treatment of Breast Cancer. *J.A.M.A.*, Nov. 18, 1988. Vol. 260, No. 19, p. 2834–2835.
128. Spratt, John S. and Greenberg, Richard A., Validity of the Clinical Alert on Breast Cancer. *The American Journal of Surgery*, 1990, Vol. 159, p. 195–198.
129. Kuehn, P. G. et al., Tissue Specificity in Multiple Primary Malignancies. *Am. J. of Surgery*, 1965, Vol. 3, No. 2, p. 164–167.
130. Storm, H. H. and Jensen, O. M., Risk of contralateral breast cancer in Denmark 1943–80, *Br. J. Cancer*, 1986, 54:483–492.
131. Urban, J. A.; Papachristou, D.; Taylor, J., Bilateral Breast Cancer. Biopsy of the opposite breast. *Cancer*, 1977, 40:1968–1973.
132. Leis, H. P., Managing the remaining breast. *Cancer*, 1980, 46:1026–1030.
133. Wanebo, H. J.; Senofsky, G. M.; Fechner, R. E.; Kaiser, D.; Lynn, S.; Paradies, J., Bilateral breast cancer. Risk reduction by contralateral biopsy. *Ann. Surg.* 1985, 201:667–677.
134. Fisher, E. R.; Fisher, B.; Sass, R. et al., Pathological Findings from the National Surgical Adjuvant Breast Project (Protocol No. 4). XI. Bilateral breast cancer. *Cancer*, 1984, 54:3002–3011.
135. Slack, N. H.; Brass, J. D.; Nemoto, T.; Fisher, B., Experiences with bilateral primary carcinoma of the breast. *Surg. Gynecol. Obstet.*, 1973, 136:433–440.

136. Martin, J. K., Jr.; van Heerden, J. A.; Gaffey, T. A., Synchronous and metachronous carcinoma of the breast. *Surgery* 1982; 91:12–16.

137. Fracchia, Alfred A.; Robinson, David; Legaspi, Adrian; Greenall, Michael J.; Kinne, David W.; Groshen, Susan, Survival in Bilateral Breast Cancer. *Cancer*, 1985, 55:1414–1421.

138. Moffat, Frederick L.; Ketcham, Alfred S.; Robinson, David S.; Legaspi, Adrian; Irani, Hormuz, Breast Cancer: Management of the Opposite Breast. *Oncology* Nov. 1988, p. 25–30.

139. Prior, P.; Waterhouse, J. A. H., Incidence of bilateral tumors in a population-based series of breast cancer patients. 1. Two approaches to an epidemiological analysis. *Br. J. Cancer* 1978, 37:620–634.

140. Robbins, G. F. and Berg, J. W., Bilateral primary breast cancer. A prospective clinicopathological study. *Cancer*, 1964, 17:1501–1527.

141. Egan, R. L., Bilateral breast carcinomas. Role of mammography. *Cancer*, 1976, 38:931–938.

142. Hislop, T. G.; Elwood, J. M.; Coldman, A. J.; Spinelli, J. J.; Worth, A. S.; Ellison, L. G., Second primary cancers of the breast: Incidence and risk factors. *Br. J. Cancer* 1984, 49:79–85.

143. Harvey, E. B. and Brinton, L. A., Second cancer following cancer of the breast in Connecticut, 1935–1982. *N.C.I. Monogr.* 1985, 68:99–112.

144. Hankey, B. F.; Curtis, R. E.; Naughton, M. D.; Boice, J. D.; Flannery, J. T., A retrospective cohort analysis of second breast cancer risk for primary breast cancer patients with an assessment of the effect of radiation therapy. *J.N.C.I.* 1983, 70:797–804.

145. Basco, V. E.; Coldman, A. J.; Elmwood, J. M.; Young, M. E. J., Radiation dose and second breast cancer. *Br. J. Cancer* 1985, 52:319–325.

146. Land, C. E.; Boice, J. D.; Shore, R. E.; Norman, J. E.; Tokunaga, M., Breast cancer risk from low-dose exposures to ionizing radiation: Results of parallel analysis of three exposed populations of women. *J.N.C.I.*, 1980, 65:353–376.

147. Ross, R. K.; Paganini-Hill, A.; Gerkins, V. R.; Mack, T. M.; Pfeffer, R.; Arthur, M.; Henderson, B. E., A case control study of menopause estrogen therapy and breast cancer. *J.A.M.A.* 1980, 243:1635–1639.

148. Cutler, S. J. and Young, J. L. (eds.) *Third National Cancer Survey Incidence Data* National Cancer Institute Monograph 41. Government Printing Office, 1975.

149. Bergkvist, Leif; Adami, H.; Perssom, I.; Hoover, R.; Schairer, C., The Risk of Breast Cancer After Estrogen and Estrogen-Progestin Replacement. *New Eng. J. Med.* Aug. 3, 1989. Vol. 321, No. 5, p. 293–297.

150. Lucas, W. E., Causal relationships between endocrine-metabolic variables in patients with endometrial carcinoma. *Obstet-Gynecol. Survey* 1974, 29:507.

151. Cutts, J. H.; Nobel, R. L., Estrone-induced mammary tumors in the rat. *Cancer Res.* 1964, 24:1116–1123.

152. Antunes, C. M. F.; Stolley, P. D.; Rosenhein, M. B. et al., Endometrial cancer and estrogen use. Report of a large case control study. *New Eng. J. Med.* 1979, 300:9.

153. Gray, L. A., Jr.; Christopherson, W. M.; Hoover, R., Estrogens and endometrial cancer. *Obstet. Gynecol.* 1977, 49:385.

154. Jelovk, F. R.; Hammond, C. B.; Woodward, B. H. et al., Risks of exogenous estrogen therapy and endometrial cancer. *Am. J. Obstet. Gynecol.* 1980, 137:85.

155. Jick, H.; Watkins, R. N.; Hunter, J. R. et al., Replacement estrogens and endometrial cancer. *New Eng. J. Med.*, 1979, 300:218.

156. Brinton, L. A.; Hoover, R.; Fraumeni, J. F., Jr., Menopausal estrogen and breast cancer risk: An expanded case-control study. *Br. J. Cancer*, 1986; 54:825–32.

157. La Vecchia, C.; Decarli, A.; Parazzini, F.; Gentile, A.; Liberati, C.; Franceschi, S., Non-contraceptive estrogens and risk of breast cancer in women. *Int. J. Cancer*, 1986; 38:853–8.

158. Hulka, Barbara, S., Hormone-Replacement Therapy and the Risk of Breast Cancer. *CA-A Cancer Journal for Clinicians*, 1990, Vol. 40, No. 5, p. 289–296.

159. Pike, M. C.; Henderson, B. E.; Krailo, M. D.; Duke, A., Breast cancer in young women and use of oral contraceptives: Possible modifying effect of formulation and age at use. *Lancet*, 1983, II:926.

160. Lincoln, R., The pill, breast and cervical cancer and the role of progestogen in arterial disease. *Family Planning Perspectives*. March–April 1984, Vol. 16, No. 2.

161. British Study Links Oral Contraception to Breast Cancer. *Oncology & Biotechnology News*, 1989, Vol. 3, No. 6.

162. Olson, H., Study finds women who took pill as teens face higher cancer risk. *The Journal Inquirer*. May 23, 1989.

163. Romieu, I.; Willett, W. C.; Colditz, G. A.; Stampfer, M. J.; Rosner, B.; Hennekens, C. H.; Speizer, F. E., Prospective Study of Oral Contraceptive Use and Risk of Breast Cancer in Women. *J. N.C.I.* 1989, Vol. 81, 17:1313–1321.

164. Ferguson, D. J. P. and Anderson, T. J., Morphological evaluation of cell turnover in relation to the menstrual cycle in the resting human breast. *British J. of Cancer*, 1981, 44·177.

165. Grattarola, R., Anovulation and increased andregenic activity as breast cancer risk in women with fibrocystic disease of the breast. *Cancer Res.* 1978, 38:3051–4.

166. MacMahon, B.; Cole, P.; Lin, T. M. et al., Age at first birth and breast cancer risk. Bull. *W.H.O.* 1970, 43:209–21.

167. Drife, J. O., Breast cancer, pregnancy and the pill. *British Med. J.*, Sept. 19, 1981, 283:778–779.

168. Brinton, L. A.; Vessey, M. P.; Flavel, R. et al., Risk factors for benign breast disease. *Amer. J. Epidmiol.* 1981, 113(3)203–14.

169. Greenspon, A. R.; Hatcher, R. A.; Moore, M. et al., "The association of depomedroxyprogestrone acetate and breast cancer." *Contraception* 1980, 21(6):563–9.

170. Bazel, U. S., "Estrogen Therapy for Osteoporosis: Is It Effective?" *Hospital Practice*. July 15, 1990, p. 95–108.

171. Watts, Nelson B.; Harris, Steven T.; Genant, Harry, K.; Wasnich, Richard D.; Miller, Paul D.; Jackson, Rebecca, D.; Licata, Angelo, A.; Ross, Philip; Woodson, Grattan, C. III; Yanover, Melissa J.; Mysiw, W. J.; Kohse, Larry; Rao, M. B.; Steiger, Peter; Richmond, Bradford; Chesnut, Charles H. III., Intermittent Cyclical Etidronate Treatment of Postmenopausal Osteoporosis. *New Eng. J. Med.* July 12, 1990, Vol. 323, No. 2.

172. Riggs, B. L.; Hodgson, Stephen F.; O'Fallon, W. M.; Chao, Edmund Y. S.; Wahner, Heinz W.; Muhs, Joan M.; Cedel, Sandra L.; Melton, L. J. III, Effect of Fluoride Treatment on the Fracture Rate in Postmenopausal Women with Osteoporosis. *New Eng. J. Med.*, March 22, 1990.

173. Silverstein, M. J.; Handel, N.; Gamagami, P.; Warsiman, J. R.; Gierson, E. D.; Rosser, R. J.; Steyskal, R.; Colburn, W., Breast Cancer in Women After Augmentation Mammoplasty. *Arch. Surg.*, 1988, Vol. 123, p. 681–685.

174. Deck, K. B.; Kern, W. H., Local recurrence of breast cancer. *Arch. Surg.* 1976, 111:323–325.

175. Cronin, T.; Gerow, F. J., Augmentation mammoplasty; a new natural feel prosthesis. In: Transactions of the third International Congress of Plastic Surgery. Excerpta Medica Foundation, Amsterdam, 1963.

176. Snyderman, R. K.; Guthrie, R. H., Reconstruction of the female breast following radical mastectomy. *Plastic and Reconstructive Surgery* 1971, 47(6):565–567.

177. d'Este, S., La technique de L'amputation de La mammelle pour carcinome mammairre. *Rev. Chir.* 1912, 45:164.

178. Davis, H. H.; Tollman, P.; Brush, J. H., Huge chondrosarcoma of rib. Report of a case. *Surgery*, 1949, 26:699.

179. Orticochea, M., The musculo-cutaneous flap method: An immediate and heroic substitute for the method of delay. *Br. J. Plastic Surg.* 1972, 25:106.

180. Radovan, C., Breast reconstruction after mastectomy using the temporary expander. *Plas. Reconstr. Surgery* 1982, 69:195.

181. Becker, H., Breast reconstruction using an inflatable breast implant with detachable reservoir. *Plastic and Reconstr. Surg.* 1984, 73(4):678–683.

182. Arnold, P. G.; Hartrampf, C. R.; Jurkiewicz, M. J., One stage reconstruction of the breast using the transposed greater omentum. *Plast. and Reconstr. Surg.* 1976, 57:520–522.

183. Robbins, T. H., Rectus abdominis myocutaneous flap for breast reconstruction. *Aust. N.Z. J. Surg.* 1979, 49:527.

184. Dinner, M. I.; Labandter, H. P.; Dowden, R. V., The role of the rectus abdominis myocutaneous flap in breast reconstruction. *Plastic Reconstr. Surg.* 1982, 69(2):209.

185. Dinner, M. I.; Dowden, R. V.; Scheflan, M., Refinements in the use of the transverse abdominal island flap for postmastectomy reconstruction. *Am. Plast. Surg.*, 1983, 11:362–372.

186. Biggs, T. M. and Cromin, E. D., Technical aspects of the latissimus dorsi myocutaneous flap in breast construction. *Ann. Plast. Surg.*, 1981, 6:381–388.

187. Shaw, W. W., Breast reconstruction by superior gluteal microvascular free flaps without silicone implants. *Plast. Reconstr. Surg.*, 1983, 72:490–501.

188. Rose, J. H., Jr., Carcinoma in a transplanted nipple. *Arch. Surg.* 1980, 115:1131–1132.

189. Cucin, R. L.; Gastos, J. P., Implantation of breast cancer in a transplanted nipple: A plea for pre-operative screening. *CA. A Cancer Journal for Clinicians.* 1981, 31(5):281–283.

190. Bartlett, W., An anatomical substitute for the female breast. *Ann. Surg.* 1917, 66:208.

191. Selye, H., A syndrome produced by diverse nocuous agents. *Nature* (Lond.) 1936, 138:32.

192. Paget, J. *Surgical Pathology, 2nd ed.* London: Longmans Green, 1870, p. 800.

193. Guy, R., *An Essay on Scirrhous Tumors and Cancers.* Churchill, London (1759). Cited on Goldfarb D.; Driesen, J.; and Cole, D., Psycholphysiologic aspects of malignancy. *Am. J. Psychiat.* 1967, 123, 1545.

194. Paget, S., The distribution of secondary growths in cancer of the breast. *The Lancet.* 1889, p. 571–73.

195. Cole, W. H., Spontaneous regression of cancer. The metabolic triumph of the host. *Ann. N.Y. Acad. Sci.* 1974, 250:111–141.

196. Keller, S. E.; Loachim, H. L.; Pearse, T.; Siletti, D. M., Decreased T-lymphocytes in patients with mammary cancer. *Amer. J. Clin. Path.* 1976, 65:445–449.

197. Cheema, A. R.; Hersh, E. M., Patient survival after chemotherapy and its relationship to in vitro lymphocyte blastogenesis. *Cancer*, 1971, 28:851–855.

198. Dilman, V. M., Metabolic immunodepression which increases the risk of cancer. *Lancet*, Dec. 10, 1977, 1207–1209.

199. Mertin, J. and Hunt, R., *Proc. Nat. Acad. Sci.* 1976, 73:928.

200. Temin, H. M., *J. Cell. Comp. Physiol.* 1969, 74:9.

201. Dilman, V. M. and Bobrov, J. F., *Sovremennze Problemi Oncologil*; 1966, p. 76. Leningrad.

202. Styjernsward, J.; Jondal, M.; Vanky, F.; Wigzell, H.; Sealy, R., Lymphopenia and change in distribution of human B & T lymphocytes in peripheral blood induced by irradiation for mammary cancer. *Lancet*, 1972, 1:1352–1356.

203. Hoover, R. and Fraumeni, J. F., Jr., Risk of cancer in renal transplant recipients. *Lancet*, 1973, 2:55–57.

204. Penn, I., Second malignant neoplasms associated with immunosuppressive medications. *Cancer*, 1976, 37:1024–1032.

205. MacMahan, B.; Cole, P.; Brown, J., Etiology of human breast cancer: A review. *J. Nat'l Cancer Inst.*, 1973, 50:21–42.

206. Armstrong, B. and Doll, R., Environmental factors and cancer incidence and mortality in different countries with special reference to dietary practices. *Int. J. Cancer*, 1975, 15:617–631.

207. Hirayanna, T., Changing pattern of cancer in Japan with special reference to the decrease in stomach cancer mortality. *H.H. Hiatt*, 1977, p. 55–75.

208. Watson, J. D. and Winsten, J. A. eds., *Origins of human cancer, book A. Incidence of cancer in humans.* Cold Spring Harbor Laboratory, Cold Spring Harbor, N.Y.

209. Dunn, J. E., Jr., Breast cancer among American-Japanese in the San Francisco Bay area. *Nat'l. Cancer Inst. Monogr.*, 1977, 47:157–160.

210. *Diet, Nutrition and Cancer*, National Academy Press, 1982.

211. *Diet and Health*, National Academy Press, 1989.

212. Pauling, L., Vitamin C therapy of advanced cancer. *N. Eng. J. Med.*, 1980, 302:694.

213. Cameron, E. and Pauling L., Supplemental ascorbate in the supportive treatment of cancer; prolongation of survival times in terminal human cancer. *Proc. Nat'l Acad. Sci. U.S.A.*, 1976, 73:3685–9.

214. Moertel, C. G.; Feming, T. R.; Creagan, E. T.; Rubin, J.; O'Connell, M. J.; Awes, M. M., High dose vitamin C versus placebo in the treatment of patients with advanced cancer who have had no prior chemotherapy. *New Eng. J. Med.*, 1985, 312:137–41.

215. Minton, J. P.; Foecking, M. K.; Webster, D. J. T.; Matthews, R. H., Caffeine, cyclic nucleotides, and breast disease. *Surgery.* 1979, 86:105.

216. Minton, J. P.; Foecking, M. K.; Webster, D. J. T.; Matthews, R. H., Response of fibrocystic disease to caffeine withdrawal and correlation of cyclic nucleotides with breast disease. *Am. Obstet. Gynec.*, 1979, 135:157.

217. Rosenberg, L.; Slone, D.; Shapior, S., Breast cancer and alcohol beverage consumption. *Lancet*, 1982, i:267–71.

218. Begey, C. B.; Walker, A. M.; Wessen, B.; Zelen, M., Alcohol consumption and breast cancer. *Lancet*, 1983, i:293–94.

219. World Health Organization 1964. Cancer agents that surround us. *World Health*, 1964, (Sep.):16–17.

220. Corrigan, J. J., Jr., and Marcus, F. I., Coagulopathy associated with vitamin E ingestion. *J.A.M.A.* 1974, 230:1300.

221. Corrigan, J. J., Jr. and Ulfers, L. L., Effect of vitamin E on prothrombin levels in a warfarin induced vitamin K deficiency. *Amer. J. Clin. Nutr.* 1981, 34:1701.

222. McGuire, R., Vitamin D Deficiency Linked to Three or Four Top Cancers. *Oncology Times*, Oct. 1990. p. 22–23.

223. Shah, J. P.; Urban, J. A., Full thickness chest wall resection for recurrent breast carcinoma involving the bony chest wall. *Cancer*, 1975, 35:567–573.

224. Jordan, V. Craig, Role of Tamoxifen in the Long-term Treatment and Prevention of Breast Cancer. *Oncology*. Sept. 1988, Vol. 2, No. 9. p. 19–26.

225. Simonton, O. C., *Getting Well Again*. Los Angeles: J. P. Tarcher, 1978.

226. Rollin, Betty, *First You Cry*. New York: Signet, 1977.

227. Kuehn, P. G., *Quality of Survival of the Cancer Patient*, Hartford Unit, American Cancer Society publication, 1969.

228. Hippocrates, Works edited by Jones W. H. and Withington, E. T., 4 volumes. New York: Putnam 1923–1931.

229. Cooper, W. A., The History of the Radical Mastectomy. *Ann. Med. Hist.* 1941, 3:36.

230. Lewison, E. F., The Surgical Treatment of Breast Cancer: An Historical and Collective Review. *Surgery* 1953, 34:904.

231. Ackerwecht, E. H., History and Geography of the Most Important Diseases. New York: Hafner, 1965 p. 162.

232. Power, D., History of the Amputation of the Breast to 1904. *Liverpool Med. Clin. J.* 1934–1935, 42/43:29.

233. Mansfield, C., Early Breast Cancer: Its History and Results of Treatment. In Wolsky, A. (Ed.) *Experimental Biology and Medicine: Monographs on Interdisicplinary Topics*. 1976, Vol. 5, New York: S. Karger, p. 2.

234. Breasted, J. H., The Edwin Smith Surgical Papyrus. Vol. 1, Chicago, University of Chicago Press, 1930, Case 39, p. 363; Case 45, p. 463.

235. Galen, C.; Opera, C. G.; Kuhn (Ed.) Leipzig, 1824.

236. Le Dran, H. F., Memoire auec un precis de plusieurs observations sur le cancer. *Mem. Aead. Roy, Chir*, 1757, 3:1.

237. Virchow, R., Die Cellularpathologic. Berlin: A Hirschwald, 1858.

238. Moore, C. H., On the Influence of Inadequate Operations on the Theory of Cancer. *R. Med. Chir. Soc.* 1867, 1:244.

ABOUT THE AUTHOR

PAUL G. KUEHN is a Surgical Oncologist, a graduate of Trinity College and the University of Rochester Medical School. He completed a general surgical residency at Hartford Hospital and then received a National Cancer Institute Fellowship for further studies in cancer at the Memorial Sloan Kettering Cancer Center in New York City where he was a senior resident in Surgical Oncology.

He was the Chairman of the American Cancer Society's National award-winning program, Quality of Survival of the Cancer Patient. He is a past president of the Hartford Unit of the American Cancer Society and of the Connecticut Division of the American Cancer Society and has also served as Chairman of the Cancer Commission for New England for the American College of Surgeons.

He is a past President of the New England Cancer Society.

The author of numerous articles on cancer for national medical journals and *Breast Care Options*, published in 1986, he is recognized as one of our country's leading cancer specialists.